My Mother,
Your Mother

My Mother,
Your Mother

EMBRACING "SLOW MEDICINE"—
THE COMPASSIONATE APPROACH TO
CARING FOR YOUR AGING LOVED ONES

Dennis McCullough, M.D.

HARPER

An Imprint of HarperCollins*Publishers*
www.harpercollins.com

MY MOTHER, YOUR MOTHER. Copyright © 2008 by Dennis McCullough. All rights reserved. Printed in the United States of America. No part of this book may be used or reproduced in any manner whatsoever without written permission except in the case of brief quotations embodied in critical articles and reviews. For information, address HarperCollins Publishers, 10 East 53rd Street, New York, NY 10022.

HarperCollins books may be purchased for educational, business, or sales promotional use. For information, please write: Special Markets Department, HarperCollins Publishers, 10 East 53rd Street, New York, NY 10022.

"When I'm alone—the words tripped off his tongue" from *Collected Poems of Siegfried Sassoon* by Siegfried Sassoon, copyright 1918, 1920 by E.P. Dutton. Copyright 1936, 1946, 1947, 1948 by Siegfried Sassoon. Used by permission of Viking Penguin Group (USA) Inc. World English language rights copyright Siegfried Sassoon by kind permission of the Estate of George Sassoon.

"Almost a thousand years ago, a Tibetan named Milarepa" from *The Caregiver's Book: Caring for Another; Caring for Yourself*, by James E. Miller, copyright © 2007 Willowgreen Publishing, Fort Wayne, Indiana. Reprinted with the permission of Willowgreen Publishing, www.willowgreen.com.

"Shapes" from *In the Next Galaxy*, copyright © 2002 by Ruth Stone. Reprinted with the permission of Copper Canyon Press, www.coppercanyonpress.org.

"Peace My Heart" from *The Gardener*, by Rabindranath Tagore, copyright © 1913. Reprinted by Kessinger Publishing Company, Whitefish, Montana, 2004. Not copyrighted in the United States (per Project Gutenberg—www.gutenberg.org/etext/6668).

FIRST EDITION

Designed by Cassandra J. Pappas

Library of Congress Cataloging-in-Publication Data is available upon request.

ISBN: 978-0-06-124302-8

08 09 10 11 12 DIX/RRD 10 9 8 7 6 5 4 3 2 1

To my mother, Bertha McCullough;
and my wife, Pamela Harrison

Contents

About Language

I have tried very hard to be inclusive in attributions of gender and relationship throughout this book, but for purposes of readability I've tended to use "mother," "father," and "parent." Certainly, Late-Life journeys are complex for both men and women, some with families, others dependent on friends and communities, some solely reliant on professional caregivers. This book honors all elders, female and male, and their supporters, of whatever variety, on the many pathways these final journeys take.

Preface

As a geriatrician practicing in America today, I often think about a Japanese film I saw years ago. In vivid images, it tells the story of three generations living in extreme poverty on a remote northerly island that afforded neither a doctor nor anything beyond the simplest folk remedies. Life was hard. Food was scarce. When the aging grandmother recognized it was her time to die, she broke her teeth with a stone so there could be no arguing about her eating the family's food. Reluctantly, inexorably, as the old woman weakened, her loving and dutiful son was forced to undertake the community's arduous tradition of carrying his mother on his back to the top of the steep and holy mountain where, as with generations past, she would be laid out with other frail elders to die a peaceful death by falling asleep in the freezing snow.

The climb up the mountain was long and difficult. The son's balance, strength, and grip occasionally failed. Engaged in their shared ritual, parent and child seldom spoke except to acknowledge their mutual trust and the difficulty of their task, or to encourage each other's spirit for what must be done. Sometimes they would pass by other couples, fathers and sons, mothers and daughters, who were tired and resting on the way. Once, hearing a horrifying wail, they saw a blurred form fall past them through the air—a parent violently thrown to her death by an impatient child before reaching the desired peak.

Those caring for their aging parents today find their journey up the mountain equally difficult and considerably longer, even with the ample benefits and miracles of contemporary medicine. The reasons for this modern paradox have taken me a lifetime of medical practice and personal experience to understand. Some of my conclusions I find surprising; others deeply disturbing.

RAISED ON WELFARE by my mother and grandfather in an impoverished Scandinavian-American mining community in the far Upper Peninsula of Michigan, I have always felt a keen allegiance to the underserved. In our quiet, stable household, as a fatherless boy, I was privileged at Saturday night saunas to sit with my grandfather and his friends and hear their stories of work, injury, and hard-earned wisdom, stories that taught me respect for them and their roles as community elders. As a medical student at Harvard, I enjoyed the mentorship of a caring older dean who stepped in with friendship and nurturing advice when my path diverged from those of classmates who sought to become specialists. Herman encouraged my persistence in following interests close to my heart. With a few other mavericks, I gravitated toward general practice, seeking a rotating internship that would prepare me for the wide scope of my future patients' needs. I then undertook a residency in family practice in Canada, where the proportion of specialists (25 percent) to generalists (75 percent) was just the reverse of our situation in the United States, and house calls were a regular part of a GP's work.

Over my years in family practice, I helped to bring natural childbirth to our northern New England rural area, made countless house

calls on those elders too weak to come to my office, forged relationships between our community hospital and the big academic center
nearby, taught medical students in my office, and took these students
to volunteer projects in third world clinics. For a year, I worked for
Project HOPE on a small Caribbean island, climbing narrow goat paths
to attend homebound elders. Gradually, an evolving fascination with
the characters and clinical complexities of my elder patients brought
me to become a geriatrician for an exceptional population of elders
at one of this country's premier continuing care retirement communities (CCRCs) in northern New England.

I might have been content to put aside my larger mission for the
underserved in favor of working with my finely trained medical team in
that warm and enlightened setting for the rest of my professional life
had I not been derailed by an unexpected and devastating personal illness that instantaneously changed me from a capable and experienced
caregiver to a weak and vulnerable care-receiver. My suddenly changed
situation brought me new emotional insights into disability and dependency. This limiting experience galvanized with a new urgency my
years of dedicated advocacy for the weak and impaired. Over the long
months of my own recovery, I thought a lot about the millions of families coping with the looming tsunami of elder care needs without sufficient resources or professional advocates to support them in their
work. I began to see how much these families might benefit from the
stories, successes, and lessons from my own experience.

FAMILIAR ANECDOTES AND clinical study confirm that, despite our
commonly expressed desire, life after age eighty rarely ends suddenly
and unexpectedly in our sleep. Past all the newsworthy excitement of
the latest promised medical fixes and experimental cures, there's no
getting around the inevitable necessity for physicians and families
alike to undertake the care of aged loved ones over months, or even

years, of decline and on through the actual work of dying—truly a "carry up the mountain." Without giving up hope for improvement or failing to look for ways to bring comfort and to enhance the quality of a parent's daily life, we must recognize and accept the mortal fact of aging's accelerating decline and overcome our denial of death. This fundamental awareness transforms what we do in our caregiving roles as adult children. It will also transform us within our own families.

Yet, so often today, despite intending to do the best work we can, we face a medical care system that seems to work at odds with our parents' stated desires and wishes—"to die at home," "to let go when the time comes," "to avoid the suffering I have seen my friends go through." Stories of elders' and families' distress abound.

When a neighbor found eighty-three-year-old Mrs. McNally in a coma in her home, Megan flew from the Midwest to join her brother for two weeks at their mother's side in the hospital. When a diagnosis of kidney failure (brought on by complications of medicines for arthritis and high blood pressure) put Mrs. McNally on a permanent course of dialysis, the doctors recommended that she no longer live alone. Megan quickly went out to explore nearby senior living options and found a nice assisted living facility that could provide enlarged social support for her mother. Her brother, however, who had not gone on those explorations, confused assisted living with nursing homes. Already feeling guilty for having been so removed from his mother's care, he wanted to take her to his home on the other side of the state "to care for her." As the time for discharge from the hospital fast approached and unable to spare any more time from work, brother and sister spent three frantic days "sorting, cleaning, and clearing" their family home so it could be sold. Mrs. McNally never saw her home again.

For the next two years, Mrs. McNally was looked after in her son's home by her daughter-in-law, the son having shied away from

actual caregiving. Having to maintain a twice-weekly schedule of
being taken by van for an all-day stint in the dialysis unit, Mrs.
McNally missed her home and old friends, lost the advocacy of her
old general practitioner, enjoyed feeling well "only two good days a
week," and lived a very "confined" life. Given her depression and the
family's conflicts, there never seemed to be a good time to discuss
advance directives. Then, one day while she was on the machine at
the dialysis unit, Mrs. McNally collapsed, presumably with cardiac
arrest. A slow response by the Fast Squad left her without oxygen to
the brain for some minutes. Finally resuscitated, she was put in the
ambulance for transport to the nearest hospital and suffered a second cardiac arrest and resuscitation en route. In the hospital ICU
(intensive care unit), the stricken elder was immediately put on a
ventilator, and dialysis was resumed. At the time Megan joined her
brother in the ICU, Megan felt "Mom was gone," but her brother
refused to hear any such talk, even accusing his sister of "giving up."
In the absence of formal advance directives to guide their decision-
making, the family continued in conflict for three days while Mrs.
McNally lay in the ICU and machines cleared her failed kidneys
and breathed for her. When Megan was told by a doctor friend
that kidney failure was a peaceful way to die, she questioned the
hospital policy of continuing active treatments on a completely
unresponsive patient. The hospital insisted on continuing all life
support because, as one doctor said, it might be "sued" by
angry family members if it did anything different.

Finally, Megan's husband arrived and negotiated gradually
turning down the oxygen to assess Mrs. McNally's capacity to
breathe on her own. Against a hospital concerned with liability,
the family was made to ask each day for the oxygen to be lessened.
After five days without significant change, the hospital relented,
moved the mother to a distant room, and discontinued dialysis.
By the time Mrs. McNally died, over another long five days, the

family members had come to feel they were "simply visiting a cadaver." After it was over, brother and sister were left with unspoken resentments, with anger at the hospital for failing to help them or their mother with compassionate care, with guilt for being unable to spare their mother a prolonged death, and with pain for her difficult, medicalized passing.

Such unfortunate situations have become so common and distressing that medical journals are now publishing lurid personal accounts of "failed care" for elders that are written by prominent physicians who themselves have been unable to get the nightmare of our disjointed health care system to respond to their own parents' needs. Frail elders are shuttled back and forth to the hospital. Care in hospitals, nursing homes, and other settings is often poorly supervised and inconsistent with an elder's and a family's wishes. Occasionally, having exceeded their paid-for length of stay in a hospital, elders die in an ambulance en route to another institution for care. "There is no room at the inn."

Industrialized, impersonal, disease-focused, technology-driven, operating against an avalanche of need, and in constant crisis mode, modern American medicine is in danger of losing its heart and soul. Pressures for efficiency and reimbursement plans skewed toward technological interventions routinely overrule more deeply caring and thoughtful responses to individual need. As a geriatrician, I know that the "canary in the coal mine" of our failing health care system is the present plight of the old and frail and their families. The vast machinery of modern medicine, which can be heroically invoked to save a premature baby, when visited upon an equally vulnerable and failing great-grandmother may not save her life so much as torturously and inhumanely complicate her dying.

In their recent opinion piece, "It's Time to March" (*Journal of the American Geriatric Society*), Drs. Knight Steel and T. Franklin Williams, two of the specialty's elder statesmen, urge that, since reform within the larger medical profession has failed, specialists in aging should take to the streets with the public in protest. "Fast Medicine" is running its lock-step, breakneck course, and no one in or out of the system seems to know how to put on the brakes. To maximize efficiency, doctors and nurses are always overscheduled. Taking time for listening and understanding—let alone time for interactions with families—is not paid for and hence not usually undertaken in these new corporate structures. No one, no matter how wealthy, enjoys the luxury of considered or reflective thought. Devoting time to practice preventive medicine can actually be considered fraudulent under our current diagnosis-based insurance schemes. Patients are briskly shunted off for various kinds of expensive, but "covered," technical testing or quickly put on medications based on ever-quickening decisions and standardized protocols. Emergency rooms are overrun with the needs of the uninsured, who wait until they are in crisis to seek care. Slower, older patients and their worried families are out of their depth, unshepherded in foreign surroundings. Bewildered by runaway situations, elders and their families know things are "not right." With few professionals left to turn to amid the busyness, larger and larger burdens of responsibility are placed on families who must carry their loved one up a steepening mountain alone.

Medicine and medicines are big business now, competing for GNP supremacy with the Department of Defense. Medical institutions, once largely not-for-profit, now look for "return on investment" when programs are planned, favoring the high yields of technologies over the "hands-on" human care really required for those with chronic illnesses. At the same time that the patient-centered heart and soul of medicine are being crushed by commercial constraints, the interface with modern medicine has predominated in the media. Cascades of drugs and drug advertising, premature reports of "breakthrough discoveries," and offers of treatments to magically stop aging (and many diseases) abound. No wonder our "canary in the coal mine" sentinels are doing so poorly. *No one can hear their quavering voices above the din.*

Yet the polar distances between technologies of modern medicine and the age-old practices of caring for the whole person can be over-come. I have seen it many times.

> Robert, nearing ninety and living independently with a spouse on the New England coast, encountered the ever-so-common heart problems of that stage of life and benefited from both surgery and medications over several years—modern medicine at its best. Eventually, another artery in his heart blocked, and he spiraled downhill, ending up in the regional hospital's intensive care unit. His situation was dire; he, his entire family, and his doctors felt the end was near. They all had talked and prepared for this for some time. The father's choice was to accept his death, and he requested "comfort measures only"—no more surgery; medications directed only toward the symptoms that distressed him. His doctors and the staff were understanding and supportive. His spouse and six children gathered around him in vigil, offering all the emotional, psychological, and spiritual support they could muster—for him and for one another. A family of singers, they sang him toward his death, which they expected to take place over hours or, at most, days. Surrounded by his loved ones, he drifted away.

My vision of better care for elders in late life is not a call for a nostalgic return to some imagined romantic past when the lone family doctor sat by the bedside by candlelight tending the ill. It is rather a stern and impassioned call to help families struggling to care for their aging and frail elders; to preserve quality of life even in the face of difficult and accumulating diseases; and to mend their neglect by modern health care "systems." My vision resonates with the old and oft-quoted statement of Harvard physician Dr. Francis Peabody: "The secret of the care of the patient is in caring *for* the patient." I have seen the erosion of this vital part of human caring in our institutional practice of medicine. But I know, because my own medical team has successfully done it, that medical institutions can support the head (technologies for care) and the heart (emotional, psychological, and spiritual support) if they set their priorities to truly "care for" each individual elder. Finding ways to empower elders and their families to carry out this vital work of creating high-quality care has become my mission.

AMERICANS TODAY ARE assailed by highly publicized reports of great advances in medicine while hearing private, whispered stories of family stress, increasing physical and practical burdens, and even financial despair. The largest portion of personal bankruptcies in the United States now stem from unpayable medical bills. These statistics don't even capture the situations of elders on fixed incomes who are always cutting back on something in order to pay for increasingly costly medications, uninsured parts of very expensive medical treatments, or totally uncovered costs of chronic care.

In this book, I focus on the fastest-growing group of elders, those over age eighty. This group is particularly important because at present it has more interaction with the medical system and uses more resources per capita than any other age group. And it is about to double its numbers, with a spiraling demand for health services. Diseases that once ended lives relatively quickly have been changed into chronic illness, chronic debilitation, and extended years of decline. The pressure of numbers is creating unprecedented family and societal burdens. Geriatric specialists like me who have been in the clinical trenches for years have learned that *this particular group of elders has the highest likelihood of benefiting from care that is more measured and reflective, and that actually stands back from rushed, in-hospital interventions and slows down to balance thoughtfully the separate, multiple, and complex issues of late life.*

Down the hall from where I work as a geriatric consultant at the Dartmouth Medical School, the groundbreaking research of Drs. Jack Wennberg and Elliott Fisher and others on the use of health services in our country shows that *more is not necessarily better.* It turns out that spending a lot of money in high-tech medical care institutions in Miami or New York City doesn't necessarily secure your mother a better outcome than the spare attentions she might get in South Dakota or Maine. How then is a family to decide what's in Grandma's (and everyone else's) best interests? The professional perspective that I bring to these pages is clinically based in traditional scientific medicine, reliant on humanistic values, and receptive to the claims and advances of complementary and alternative therapies. It reflects my thirty years in community medical practice capped by a decade's experience shaping the health care philosophy and practice of the Kendal-at-Hanover community of elders.

Members of this New Hampshire continuing care retirement community (average age eighty-four) used resources wisely to create the health care system they wanted. The proximity of my clinical geriatric practice to one of the United States' highest-rated academic medical centers, the Dartmouth-Hitchcock Medical Center, makes superior technical medical care easily available and keeps our elder community very alert to the latest advances in medical science. Yet the wisdom of this community of retirees—former Rhodes scholars, college presidents, many with academic and professional backgrounds (many are retired physicians)—is grounded in a Yankee conservatism that refuses to accept, carte blanche, all high-tech claims. Without any sacrifice of satisfaction, this cautious conservatism, supported by the steady attentions of our Kendal health care team working with families, results in health care of unusually high and sustaining quality. In fact, our recent studies of end-of-life care show expenditures for our patients to be *far less* than expenditures for a matched senior group getting "standard care" in our academic medical center.

Families must come to appreciate that "medicalized" care is very different in nature and cost from the personal health support and hands-on caring so essential for your parent. In reality, our American medical system is best at managing acute crises and supplying excellent specialized elective procedures—joint replacements, organ transplants, eye improvements, cosmetic changes—all modern technological wonders. As for the more ordinary and common management and support of elders and families dealing with chronic problems of aging and slow-moving diseases, our medical care system has not done so well. Some elderly patients are fruitlessly subjected to what some critics now call "death by intensive care"—that is, sedated and thus unable to communicate; enduring impersonal medical protocols in strange, disorienting surroundings; or stranded in limbo on life-support machines while families hover in waiting rooms, uncertain how to help.

This high drama happens for some, but much more commonly in my experience elders suffer the accumulating burdens of illness and exhausting medical regimens that extract available energies and time, leaving nothing left for living beyond a "medicalized" life. But there is another way, a family-centered, less expensive way shaped by habits of cooperation, coordination, and conservation of limited resources. This is what I call Slow Medicine, and it can be practiced by you, your family, and all those who will attend your parent during his or her "journey up the mountain."

Slow Medicine is a special commitment undertaken by families and health professionals working together to achieve the *very fullest understanding* of aging loved ones and their complex, ever-evolving needs. This, in turn, leads to wiser decision-making regarding formal medical interventions. There are specific strategies and approaches for making life better for elders and their families. The journey with our loved ones through the final decades of their lives should not be strewn with wasted opportunities and complicated by the wrong kind of medicine.

Far from the cinematic drama of hospital emergency rooms, *Slow Medicine embraces the unsung work of daily attention that is the greatest need and firmest foundation for longevity and quality of life at the farthest reach of age.* Excellent chronic care attends to the day-to-day needs and conditions of the patient—by offering emotional support and social stimulation, supplying better nutrition, easing chronic skin and nail conditions, and making sleeping, moving, bathing, dressing, and voiding easier. Slow Medicine is the careful practice that most reliably sustains fragile patterns of well-being. This foundation for better elder care strengthens, rather than replaces, the selective use of high-tech care.

During the time of the writing of this book, I have lived the story of my own mother's decline in health in a very different setting. The rural Upper Peninsula of Michigan shares one characteristic with the region around Dartmouth-Hitchcock: a very high percentage of older folks in its population. Dartmouth is a magnet for well-to-do retirees; the U.P. is a reservoir of poor elders left behind by young people moving away to seek work. For a doctor practicing around Dartmouth, so much was available; for a son in rural Michigan, so very little. Yet the same process of the conservative middle way has served my mother in her setting as well as it has served my patients at Dartmouth in theirs.

Late Life is a specific and special time of aging, and elders and their families need to engage this time more fully, consciously, practically, and successfully. *This is not a plan for getting ready to die; it is a plan for understanding, for caring, and for living well in the time that is left.*

I've identified eight distinct stations along the path of late life and described the texture of life commonly experienced in each by elders and their families. I forewarn families of particular issues and new opportunities encountered during this journey, making suggestions for what questions to ask and what conversations to initiate. Extensive lists of practical tasks at each station provide specific counsel for engaging constructive work and change.

Using this book, you and your family can learn to advocate for better, more personal, and more responsive care for your loved ones. You can more surely shepherd your parents' and your family's emotional, physical, and financial resources along the path. You can take steps to make this shared journey more thoughtful, controlled, and rich with quality of life. And, just as I have learned as a doctor and son with my own mother, you may be strengthened and consoled, finding satisfaction and even joy through your embrace of this vital late-life work. I am confident that Slow Medicine will become the strongest foundation for your family journey.

First Things

The Foundation of a New Family Understanding

Italy is where the modern idea of slowness was born. This family-centered country first conceived the Slow Food movement to counter the invasion and industrial excesses of American fast foods. By promoting regional flavors and locally grown variety, and by taking time for conversation and digestion, they reclaimed the high quality of a basic human experience, not to mention salvaging more healthful nutrition for their citizens. Later, the Italians extended the concept to their urban environments, designating Slow Cities, where automobiles were banned from central plazas, helping grandmothers to be safe and welcome on the streets.

I've adopted this idea of slowness to benefit this special population of Late-Life elders who do not move or think as swiftly, see or hear as clearly; whose health problems and solutions are more complex; whose energy stores and resilience are less; and whose recovery takes more time than for us at middle age. Slow Medicine's ultimate goal is a practical and qualitative change in care directed by a more complete respect for and fuller understanding of the particularity of each late-life elder.

This practice calls for *using the allotted time health professionals (and families) spend with our aging parents differently and making better, more appropriate decisions more slowly and over a more extended period of time.* Doing this work well cannot be reduced to knee-jerk routines. It requires more thoughtful evaluation and reflection, attentive listening, looking, and hands-on participation. It also demands that we ask for medical care different from what most elders are presently allowed: the fifteen-minute office call to renew prescriptions while the doctor peers into a computer screen or the answering machine's advice to go to the emergency room. No sound bite distillations of information entered into a prefabricated electronic flow sheet can elicit or make sense of the complexities of an elder's needs, unspoken concerns, and nuances of illness at these nether reaches of age. Focusing on blood pressure control without knowing the patient well enough or talking long enough to recognize subtle losses of cognition and strength doesn't get to the heart of the patient's (or the family's) real problems. Knowing the daily burdens, emotional demands, and psychological intricacies of your mother's days in her apartment can't be undertaken by her doctor alone. Slow Medicine requires intimacy and commitment on the part of many others. The best care results when health care professionals, family members, and caregivers share information. These conversations allow discoveries and responses to percolate within a clinician's intuition and subconscious over time, leading to a deeper understanding of an older person's present situation and the future.

These balanced, mutually respectful, and supportive partnerships between doctors, nurses, and other health professionals and elder patients, their families, close friends, neighbors, and anyone else chosen to be part of what I call the Circle of Concern are at the heart of Slow Medicine. This group of people who naturally connect to a person in trouble provides steady support and insight. Although at middle age we might engage the help of such a group for a sudden crisis, for failing elders the Circle of Concern gathers for the long run. This active, extended advocacy partnership can improve our elders' care by attending to both technical and human needs, and by balancing the formal care from professionals and institutions with a particular individual's physical, emotional, and financial capacities, family values, and personal philosophical or spiritual outlook. Tailoring such extended and personalized care for a former waitress will be different from tailoring care that might suit a retired college dean—neither is simply "a white-haired old lady."

Slow Medicine is not really new in the annals of medicine, but it needs to be retrieved and given prominence again. Many doctors in the trenches are in mourning for the age-old practice of paying deep attention and truly "attending" that is being squeezed from our complex, fragmented, and technological medical system. Slow Medicine for elders in late life enacts the ancient Tibetan wisdom of "making haste slowly," that is, focusing on the central issues of human caring with patience and a sense of shared humanity, forgiving one another for what cannot be changed, bending flexibly at times of need, and holding firmly to shared values and loyalties at other times. Slow Medicine is a commitment to understand, to support, to heal, and to care for those weakest among us in a way we would want to be cared for ourselves.

Over my many years of medical practice, I have identified five fundamental principles that should guide families, health professionals, caregivers, and other caring people in their efforts to enrich and support an elder's life to the end.

I. We must endeavor to understand our parents and other elders deeply, in all their personal complexity, acknowledging both the losses and the newly revealed strengths that come with aging.

Shortly before her death at ninety-two, Agnes talked about "closing the circle." Having grown up in the South in a prominent Georgia family, she knew and loved her family history. To Agnes, "passing on" was simply what a person did. You passed on from your own life, and you passed on the role you held in your family to those who came after. What a clear sense she enjoyed of how her individual life fit into a long-recorded and remembered family history! The colorful stories told after her passing made her special qualities very clear.

As we mature, our culture encourages us to become fully who we are, to realize our personal potential, and evolve as unique individuals. We also come to recognize that though our individual lives are as miraculously detailed and unique as snowflakes, they can just as easily be obscured in a blizzard of others. From birth to death, we experience our life's passage as highly personal, but just as surely our span of years conforms to the limits and possibilities of our human species. There is the truth of highly individualized experience, and there is the very different truth of statistical patterns. We shouldn't be surprised when families and medical science take differing perspectives on aging, illness, and death. A heart specialist is trained to focus on your mother's loss of heart muscle strength (her "congestive heart failure"); your family, on the other hand, must focus on what this change means for her chances of living alone in her home each day and what emotional, mental, and spiritual concerns arise as a consequence of her new physical limitations.

As we age, our individuation becomes ever more distinct. Biologically and genetically determined characteristics, personality traits and types, character development, and life experience—all these influences enter into the complex process of becoming a particular person. The artist began doodling in his schoolbook and increasingly grew more singular and adept with time and experience; similarly the teacher, the salesman, and the secretary. Over the years, all the various ways we operate and habits we develop establish unique patterns. These are not only patterns of behavior and habit, but also *actual neuron pattern and functioning differences set down in our brains.* We should not be surprised then by just how unique each human being has become by late life.

As a parent or friend ages and encounters illness, disability, and decline, his or her family and caregivers must always strive to see the person first when considering health care needs and decisions. The experience of rehabilitation after knee surgery for an older athlete will be very different from that for a retired bus driver. We must also see each unique life in the larger, more general context of the "closing circle." In the end, for all of us, death prevails. We need to see our parents in all their complexity while at the same time striving to do what is best at each station on the road of Late Life. For every parent, every elder, as losses accumulate, so often strengths—particularly emotional and spiritual strengths—emerge. As we journey together down the road, looking for and working with a parent's new capacities—such as newly found humor, acceptance, resolve, or patience—is the challenge for health care and family caring.

II. We must accept the need for interdependence, while at the same time promoting mutual trust.

> "No," Carlotta explained to her sixty-five-year-old son. "Your Aunt Maria lives right next door and can always come by if I need her." The conversation was coming to its familiar end. He knew since childhood how stubborn his mother could be and how she continued to triumph over reason. She had shrunk to four feet, nine inches, but her power remained. How could a "couple" of falls and a night on the floor deter her? The ambulance returned her to her lifelong home, and, by her own estimation, she was "doing fine." She had won again. Would the family and neighbors all lose as a result? He wasn't sure that this was the right decision. Next month, they would talk it all over again—on Aunt Maria's eighty-ninth birthday.

"Holding out," usually alone or perhaps with a compliant spouse, is a common response to aging for many people, no matter their social standing or economic class. "We can take perfectly good care of ourselves." "I'll tell you when I need you." "I'm not leaving this house." Holding out may have its roots in stubborn American individualism. We don't like to admit the need for help. Dependency rankles. Our parents want to maintain their customary freedom and autonomy. Perhaps it's a financial matter: they don't want to be a drain on their children. Or perhaps resistance to change flows from an informed fear of the local nursing home. Elders' families and friends need to see this preference as a logical response to the circumstances of Late Life, when mental, physical, and emotional capacities are diminishing.

At the same time, holding out, as legitimate and even admirable as it may feel while it is going well, in many ways encourages a sudden and rapid turn to its opposite. Aging parents (often viewed as "stubborn") may resist interventions until things fall apart, as they almost always do. Then, adult children (or close friends or neighbors or social workers or health professionals) have to move in to take over. *Holding out seldom promotes the shared autonomy and give-and-take rhythms and practice of Slow Medicine that allow the optimal maintenance of independence while still meeting the changing needs that inevitably arise.*

On the other hand, jumping in is the wrong strategy as well. Adult children coming to this book because of emerging issues for their parents must first do their own preparatory work. In the prime of your life, in possession of superior understanding and practical capabilities, you may feel prepared to engage many of the problems your parents face more effectively than they can themselves. Indeed, you may think it would be both uncaring and irresponsible not to do so. Slow down. Walk a day in their shoes. Many elders have suffered the unexpected consequences of an unsolicited intrusion. *Instigating single-handed solutions may in fact destroy the mutual trust that is the best foundation for the work ahead.*

Dependency is difficult for most adults and feels particularly sham-ing for the strongest and most accomplished of us when it comes on unexpectedly. Although growing old may be an essential fact of life, no amount of mental preparation can really help us to understand what we face with disability and aging and what it feels like to be forced, af-ter years of unquestioned autonomy, to rely on the help of family and utter strangers. Likewise, adult children, after enjoying some decades of autonomous adulthood and lately graduated from the rigors of rais-ing their own children, may be shocked to have to enter again into an active interdependency with an aging parent.

The balance between autonomy and supportive intervention is com-plex. Just as the teenager must learn to practice autonomy, the parents must learn to trust and support their child's judgments. When the situ-ation and one's sense of parental responsibility call for it, trust must be balanced by the need for some degree of intervention. This is a dif-ficult dynamic to learn and may entail some failures while all those involved refine their skills. Human relationships at the far end of the life cycle are similarly difficult, and the skills for managing these rela-tionships are equally taxing to learn. This is true for both parent and adult child. One isn't naturally skilled at this give-and-take. It is a learned activity.

The practice of Slow Medicine has taught me that it is wise to slow down and moderate the urgent pressures of decision-making that are often pushed prematurely on elders by society, the medical profession, worried friends, and family. Well-intentioned, we want to make good and humane choices for ourselves and for those we love. We are trou-bled by guilty feelings of neglect if we wait too long to act. We often experience nagging doubts of our adequacy in these new and very changed relationships. We live in a society of increasingly tight sched-ules and pressure-filled, assembly-line efficiencies. We are conditioned to want the maximum application of resources, and we are drawn to the latest technologies rather than humble, slow, old-fashioned, labor-intensive hands-on work. We are being asked to choose video surveillance of our parents' homes over regular telephone calls and visits and telemedicine home monitoring of weight and blood pressure over neighborly companionship.

I cannot emphasize enough that the years of Late Life can seldom be managed neatly or even adequately through approaches that led to success in people's younger years. Insisting on efficiency, promoting multitasking rather than careful listening and being "in the moment," and ignoring the needs for slower transitions during times of change in our parents' lives serve neither them nor us. We want our parents at all times to feel that they are fully understood. This will not be easy when they are in a stage of life sometimes marked by lost capacities of insight and communication. This special time of heightened interdependency requires solutions that emerge out of established and engaged relationships, hard-achieved consensus, and mature understanding. The achievement of mutual trust is as important as any work of early family building and child rearing and one of the surest hopes for ameliorating the pain and sadness of loss.

III. We must learn to communicate well and with patience.

All six children and even the grandchildren wrote in Sarah's "diary" whenever they came to visit her in the nursing home. Recorded were the simple activities they each undertook with Grammie during their visits. Each family member also wrote notes detailing discussions with the supervising floor nurse and Grammie's "real nurses," particularly Jasmine, the nursing aide, who was their elder's favorite and knew the most about her. During Sarah's slow decline, the notes helped the family navigate, each note correcting course, showing how variably her life winds blew from day to day. And later, these saved notes helped to sustain the memories of her life and their commitment, softening their grieving.

Language, both spoken and nonverbal, can enhance or distort reality. Good communication is a foundation for the success of any venture and especially for any relationship that must face change and the unexpected challenges of sudden crises. No matter how many resources you and your family may have ready and waiting to exercise on your loved ones' behalf, if you or the organization you are dealing with has poor, sporadic methods of communicating accurate logistic, physical, and emotional details, your parents will not receive the care he or she deserves. Communication between different care settings may be altogether lacking. Medical and institutional jargon may be incomprehensible to the uninitiated. Good communication requires awareness that different groups use the same words to mean different things—and poorly chosen actions may override the best-chosen words.

Good communication requires the willingness to listen to what is actually said, to take notes and ask questions—and also to recognize that there may be much that remains *unsaid out of fear, confusion, haste, or uncertainty.* Communication, as all diplomats and married couples know, is a difficult art that requires great tact, patience, repeated clarifications, and continual practice. Honed communication skills are absolutely essential to the successful practice of Slow Medicine.

IV. We need to make a covenant for steadfast advocacy.

Elaine's son flew in from California and arrived at the hospital just as the gathered family members were heading home and feeling relief at having finally reached consensus through extended and sometimes difficult conversations among themselves and with Elaine's physicians. While the rest of the family agreed on pursuing a less aggressive approach to Elaine's failed chemotherapy, their prodigal sibling, alarmed, armed with stories offered by friends and work colleagues on the other coast, and anxious to make up for his absence, insisted on another detailed review of the whole situation.

Tired, but resigned, the family and Elaine's personal physician gathered again the next day for the work to be done.

Mobility has become a defining characteristic of American life. It has caused the fragmentation of families and communities and led to the development of patterns of living that are substantially changed from those of the past. Retirees leave their larger communities and move into the geographic segregation of age-limited enclaves. Children live at considerable distances from their families of origin, complicating the work of familial care. The stability that once underwrote our communal and familial health has given way to speed and change.

At the same time, the prevalence of litigation to soften the economic effects of bad medical outcomes and the deteriorating state of continuity of care by health professionals are increasingly shifting the day-to-day responsibility for decision-making from professionals back onto families. Regional differences in approaches to medical care, local differences in the availability of out-of-hospital support services, and differing community attitudes toward care for the elderly all complicate the current process of reaching consensus on "the right thing to do."

Our medical care system as it is presently structured promotes a crisis response rather than developing (and paying for) reliable support systems to help families and individuals cope with extended chronic burdens. For elders during this Late-Life stage, predictable crisis cycles of hospital–rehabilitation–nursing home stays are often repeated many times over.

In reflecting on the decades of work I've done as a clinician, I see that my primary role might best be described as "physician friend." Ethicist William May's concept of the "covenantal relationship" is another way of thinking about this doctor-patient alliance. In such partnerships, the doctor expressly becomes the designated "agent" of the patient and family and maintains a covenant, unspoken and unwritten, to be there in time of need. This is an enormous responsibility at any time, although I imagine that it was somewhat easier to fulfill in the past when society was less mobile and medical care was less complex and specialized in its organization and delivery.

I have found that as a working practice, any covenantal relationship usually develops into a two-way commitment. Just as years of regular clinical care have afforded me a many-layered understanding of my patients' psychological, emotional, and physical circumstances, so, over time, my patients become more attuned to recognizing both their own needs in the moment and my needs as their serving "physician partner." This kind of two-way *personal and professional relationship of mutual trust* provides a strong foundation for the kind of care elders need along the road of Late Life.

Today's sophisticated medical technologies require a great deal of specialized expertise from physicians as well as timely, coordinated teamwork to deliver optimum care. In many communities throughout our country, there is a general shortage of primary care physicians to follow their patients into the hospital and reliably take on this role of personal shepherd. Despite goodwill and their instinctive desire to be helpful, supportive, and healing, most specialists and hospital doctors, nurses, and staff members (right down to those who do the most humble but important jobs in health care) feel pressured today by a medical system that stresses industrial efficiency and high productivity, making it difficult or impossible for them to perform this covenantal role. Without a guiding professional friend who has the authority to act in a range of situations and locations commonly encountered in Late Life, it is common for patients and families to flounder. In medical systems operating according to complex institutional protocols and burdened by paper-clogged shuffles among various specialists focused on particular diseases and separate parts of the body, there is no one to reliably assume the role of knowledgeable patient advocate, no one to integrate and interpret in-hospital information and services, no one to coordinate services for out-of-hospital care.

If your parent's physician cannot undertake this vital responsibility, look around among your family and friends in the community. Is there a nurse, social worker, or care manager that you might call on? Finding such a formal or informal advocate, becoming one yourself, or creating a team of advocates makes all the difference.

V. We must maintain an attitude of kindness no matter what.

The most important consideration underlying all my assumptions about what constitutes good late-life care is the need for kindness. Although some families and caregivers may actually rise to extended enactments of love (or simply loyalty, decency, respect, and gratitude), *kindness is the single most reliable ethical and practical guide to doing this work well.* Because of the ultimate powerlessness and dependency, indeed, the utter frailty of the old and infirm, kindness is the fundamental position that a caregiver has to sustain. This is not always easy.

Days of caregiving are long and difficult, and each interaction between caregiver and care-receiver requires patience and forbearance as part of a seemingly endless cycle of chores. Both at home and in institutions, the risk of mistreatment is ever present. A family member or worker with the elderly who can't assume an attitude of kindness is (or should be) a concern to any organization or family that is engaged in this work. This includes everyone, all the way up through doctors, the staff, and administrators in our hospitals and nursing homes.

———

Sam and Gladys were racing toward ninety, still together in their apartment, although now he had to push her in a wheelchair when they went out for groceries or to a restaurant. Small strokes had whittled away at her speech and judgment. Both knew the end of independence and apartment living was in sight, but given that they had three marriages between them, there were many unfamiliar children and grandchildren to involve in the decision. Together they all set off on a voyage of building trust. Over the course of a year, plans were worked through and two different sets of children operated in sequence to dismantle the household. Both groups of children sent representatives to the nursing home meeting where Sam and Gladys were debating the idea of separate rooms—she for it, he against. After group discussion, she prevailed. Twice a day, Sam collected Gladys in her wheelchair to go to the dining room together. Their journey took another three years to complete. Their deaths came six months apart, Sam unexpectedly passing first. By the end, both families had learned to advocate as one.

Over the course of the chapters ahead, we will be taking a long journey together up the challenging path of Late Life. We'll begin now with that quiet period you may look back to as a time of blessed stability.

The Eight Stations of Late Life

Stability

———∞∞∞———

"Everything is just fine, dear."
—MOM

At eighty-five my mother, Bertha, begins her morning when she wants to. No hurry to get up and out. Keep the nightgown on or gradually get dressed. (So many clothes in the closet, but fewer used.) Remember to place the placard outside on the apartment doorknob so that the administrator in her senior living complex knows that she is safely up and started. The *Daily Mining Gazette* is at the door for reading in her green chair by the window with instant coffee. Perhaps a little cold cereal later. . . . Get dressed for lunch and take a walk downstairs. Check the mail—"air mail," she calls it when the box is empty. Chat with friends and fellow "inmates" over a hot lunch. Pick up a box-dinner for eating later. Return to her room for a nap. Wake and take a long walk outdoors, weather permitting, or take the trolley to the mall and walk indoors. Choose a birthday card for one of her four great-grandchildren. Take another nap before working on the paper's crossword puzzle. Bingo this evening. The Pistons are playing later tonight. And next month, she'll be going with me to Hawaii, a lifelong dream come true that's the envy of her friends. Looks like a good day.

Like many in her Greatest Generation, my mother started life with early difficulties. Her mother died when she was eleven, forcing her, as the oldest daughter, to drop out of the village school in order to keep house and raise four younger siblings. A straight-A student and an avid reader, she has mourned the loss of an education the rest of her days. During World War II, a short-lived marriage left her alone with two young children and landed her back in the security (and limits) of the family home, caring then as well for her aging father. A sturdy constitution, good humor, good personal habits, stable living conditions, and improving luck in life (she was a regular winner of door prizes and at pinochle) blessed Bertha with excellent health but few resources when she retired from keeping house for others and stuffing sausages at the local meat plant. Apart from suffering some depression at age sixty-five when she had to leave the family home for lack of money to maintain it, she cruised through crises on a stream of cheerful stoicism and denial. Minor chronic medical difficulties—glaucoma, high blood pressure, scoliosis, osteoporosis, a little arthritis, a prolapsed uterus—and two short hospitalizations, one for a heart rhythm problem, the other a two-day stay for gallbladder surgery, had us thinking she might go on living just the way she was, forever.

STABILITY IS OUR hope—smooth sailing under white clouds and sunny skies on a July day. For the individual, the partner, the family, and indeed everyone in an elder's circle, we would love for life to go on just like this . . . forever. Who could not wish for Mother to continue to live as comfortably and well as she is living right now—eighty-five, in her own home, and being fully herself? For elders like Bertha, what value is there in fretting, worrying, or measuring where one is in the natural span of life? Self-reflection is a luxury and bother she has done without. All is well now. She has a family who cares about her and seeks her company; friends; the familiarity of an apartment where she has lived for eighteen years; a community that knows her by face and name and that enjoys a long-honored tradition of progressive care for its elders; and a regular personal physician she consults for her high blood pressure (and the odd illness, should that happen). The four (or is it really six?) medications she takes (drops for glaucoma and two she doesn't consider medicines, just "supplements"—aspirin and B$_{12}$) are a once-a-day routine that she has down pat. These are the important particulars of her life.

And particulars are what matter. For instance, your mother may have a mate, so her routine will be a little bit different. There is some reminding going on between Mom and Dad, back and forth, more or less amicably—or maybe mostly forth. ("Don't forget your eye appointment tomorrow." "You forgot to turn off the burner again." "You haven't zipped up your skirt.") Some things have slipped a little. Dad has lost some of his former sharpness. Now your parents joke openly when they talk on the phone about their outings in the car. "It's all right, dear. Dad steers and watches the left side, and I cover the right. He looks, and I listen. You know, he still refuses to wear the hearing aid. Lots of money for nothing there." Still two for the road. Proof that your parents' partnership is still strong. They have propped each other up through the bad times, and in some ways these later years do seem easier, more carefree than the past.

As for you and your siblings and your families—is there anyone you know who isn't busy and occasionally stretched too thin? Life seems to have accelerated and to be more stressful, with tighter schedules, longer work hours, more demanding expectations of performance and reward. Besides, though we may be flung to the far corners of the country and separated now by both miles and differing local cultures, our extended families are in touch as time allows—regularly by telephone, the occasional letter or postcard, and brief yearly visits. E-mail also helps many of us to maintain regular contact. All is well. We are the lucky ones. Why complicate everyone's lives with worry before it's absolutely necessary?

Why Not Let Sleeping Dogs Lie?

There is much value in quietly leaving things alone. We have learned from experience, and particularly in our extended families, that there are some subjects that are off-limits—money, sex, politics, and religion may be on your family's list, as they are my wife's. Anything to do with my mother and father's brief life together has been taboo for me and my sister. From our parents' generation's stoical perspective, it was better to skirt many issues, keeping mum about choices concerning child rearing, money, jobs. A few crises along the way may have required our families to cross these boundaries, but for the most part we are, or have been, discreet and tolerant. In our culture, we learn to respect independence, privacy, differences of opinion, and exercises of autonomy. Mostly, we have avoided imposing our thoughts and beliefs on one another.

Of course, parenting was the exception. As kids, when our parents exerted control, we didn't argue (until we needed to). Later, when we had our own kids, we valued the familial hierarchy as natural and necessary to the risks and duties of that special nurturing period of the life cycle. Now that our own kids are almost launched, we find we can begin to talk more easily and openly, sharing with them some of the horror stories of their adolescence with the good humor of distance. Perhaps you are part of a younger generation, having a family later in life, and the experience of parenting is yet to unfold fully. If this is the case, you'll surely be sandwiched between your children's and your parents' needs.

The first wave of baby boomers, members of this large sandwich generation, are only now beginning to appreciate the quickly approaching later parts of the human life cycle. As this generation's great wave of baby boomers has matured, the nation's practical interest in sociology and psychology has paralleled their aging. The rash of popular self-help books on the midlife crisis (initially for men) and the menopause years for women anticipated the boomers' own experience of those times of life. As with all work in progress, the generations to follow will refine their particular variants of the big life-cycle issues. Theories will rise and fall, but generally we are still enacting Shakespeare's view on the seven ages of man in *As You Like It* (infancy, childhood, adolescence, young adulthood, middle age, old age, senility), phases that are elemental and inescapable, but with luck and curiosity may be reflected upon, understood, and improved. Here are the last three ages, from middle age to near death.

> And then the justice
> In fair round belly with good capon lined,
> With eyes severe and beard of formal cut,
> Full of wise saws and modern instances;
> And so he plays his part. The sixth age shifts
> Into the lean and slippered pantaloon,
> With spectacles on nose and pouch on side,
> His youthful hose, well saved, a world too wide
> For his shrunk shank; and his big manly voice,
> Turning again toward childish treble, pipes
> And whistles in his sound. Last scene of all,
> That ends this strange eventful history,
> Is second childishness and mere oblivion,
> Sans teeth, sans eyes, sans taste, sans everything.

Shakespeare's Seven Ages of Man speech, written now four centuries ago, colorfully encapsulates much of our modern thinking about our human life cycle. Keep in mind that you, the "justice adult" at age forty to sixty-five, are highly empowered at this stage, while your parents may be struggling with their impending loss of power. This is the classical disparity (and often a source of conflict) in late life.

By watching and listening carefully, we may discover the model of aging that guides our parents. We like to interpret our elders' silence as denial, but in my clinical experience there are life conditions and seasons elders clearly understand and recognize, even if they are not drawn to overt analysis. Dr. Spock sold a lot of books on child rearing, and my mother missed them all. But she had very clear, if unarticulated, ideas about what constituted good parenting and appropriate care, and she practiced them day by day for years. A few pioneers in her generation may actually follow what is being written about the advanced age part of the human life cycle, but generally this older cohort does not hold the same curiosity or self-help drive that our psychology-steeped generation exhibits. Nor does that cohort share our compulsion to verbalize everything we may be experiencing.

So, why not let sleeping dogs lie? When our parents tell us, "Everything is fine, dear," why should we perk up and pay attention? And what would we pay attention to?

There is a time of relative calm before elders decline from disease, illness, accident, and aging. During this Station of Stability, however brief or long it may prove, individuals, families, health care systems, and medical professionals should actively observe, evaluate, and prepare in ways that can reduce the effects of sure-to-come future crises. By preparing for their inescapable eventuality, we can spare ourselves and our parents practical, emotional, and physical difficulty and suffering. While there is still time to act, individuals and their families must awaken to the inevitability of disruptive change, the storms after the calm that medical professionals are so accustomed to seeing in Late Life. Because even the best physician can never know when this period of relative calm and smooth sailing will end, it is best to engage this work immediately and proactively, even when things are going well.

> For the third straight year the result of the review and the exam was the same. Now in his eighties, Alan always looked forward to my summary.
>
> "You are an extraordinarily healthy man for your age. I can't say that I've found anything of concern."
>
> "That's great, Doc," he responded with a twinkle in his eye. "Do you suppose that means anything about tomorrow?"

What does an annual Slow Medicine review consist of? Unlike the battery of lab tests and screenings a doctor might order for you at middle age, in late life it is rather an exercise in attentive listening. My questions focus on medical problems certainly, but also include asking how an elderly man, say, spends his time, searching for clues about his emotional state, observing how his mind works, and inviting him to share his own insights about these important aspects of successful aging. Including interested family members later in the review almost always adds an important new dimension of understanding. Helping your parent to prepare in advance improves an "overview" visit's value. Although there are questionnaires designed to screen for depression, cognition loss, and functional change, such screening tools are often not very sensitive to the earliest changes noted by the people themselves and their families. If you participate in a visit, not only will you learn more about your parents' medical problems; you will also get to observe the doctor-patient relationship, which is always revealing—sometimes comforting, sometimes alarming.

Practical Tasks at the Station of Stability

PUT YOURSELF IN THEIR SHOES

Go Over the Events of Your Family's "Growing Up" and "Growing Older"

Remember the questions we asked back at the start of parenting our own children?

Is this normal?

What new behavior should we look for at this next stage?

What's the best way to spend our time together?

Should we have a talk with the teacher?

As we maintained a home and pursued our chosen work, often pulling up roots to follow a job, we slowly became aware that time was passing and we were becoming our parents.

I never thought I'd actually buy a suit.

Turn down that music!

You may not wear that out of the house!

Later we discovered our own middle age.

I've gained ten pounds!

I can't find my glasses.

I forgot what I came here for.

Suddenly everyone needs orthotics!

Be aware that the same changes hold true with family life-cycle stages.

The kids aren't coming home for Christmas?

You're talking just like your mother.

Son, will you please explain how this thing works?

We find ourselves living generational clichés that we discern or admit to only in retrospect. But what is different is that our longer-living parents and our later-born children are making us the sandwich generation for a longer period of time. Suddenly our energies, as well as resources, must go out both to our children (whose support we may have thought or wished we had completed with the last college tuition payment) and to our parents (with whom we are quickly and nervously getting reacquainted). The Pew Research Center recently reported that the percentage of baby boomers aged forty-one to fifty-nine who gave financial help to a parent in the last year was 29 percent and the percentage who gave financial help to an adult child was 57 percent.

Are Changes Individual or Part of a Common Aging Process?

Just as we have begun to experience uncomfortable shifts from the vigor and resilience of our youth, so our parents are passing forward into new areas of limitation and reduced competencies. How much of Mother's new (troubling) behavior is simply a playing out of the "way she has always been"? How much just comes along with the Late-Life territory? Check Appendix II and Appendix III for suggestions of books and movies of engaging stories and reflections that take us back centuries to reveal the commonness of human sentiments and emotional responses in Late Life. For example, the third century B.C.E. Chinese philosopher Chuang Tzu commented, "I received life because the time had come; I will lose it because the order of things passes on." The movie *Wrestling Ernest Hemingway* explores friendships and complex emotions in aging in the setting of a small Florida community; *About Schmidt* and *Innocence* look at the power of both loneliness and love. You may find more movies on the foreign shelves than get produced in our youth-centered culture. Remember, common human themes cut across cultures.

Learn About Aging

What exactly happens to bodies besides the weight gain and sag we so often joke about? How does a person's skeleton change with age? Men's ears get hairy and their heads bald, and Dad's eyebrows take on a life of their own. Where did Mother's eyebrows go? Doesn't she see how weird her wrinkles look under that dyed red hair? How does our gait change in Late Life? Our balance? What we can see? What we can hear? In what ways do reflexes and thinking slow down? How do these changes affect driving? When is it time to ask for the car keys? What states require relicensing for seniors? Does your parents' community have a "55 Alive" program for evaluating and brushing up driving skills? Is it a matter of Mom's driving speed or a decline in her skills? What are the mental operations that Dad is still good at? There are loads of resources out there. Start reading up. (See Appendix II.)

Discuss How Decisions Get Made

As Americans we all value our perceived right to do as we wish. "The choice of therapy is up to you," says the doctor to your mother in the last thirty seconds of her allotted time. But is the choice really up to her? Is she being given adequate time through Slow Medicine practice to ponder or seek additional advice, or is she being "guided" too quickly toward a course of action? What is such a rushed judgment worth to an elder who thinks and talks and understands more slowly? Maybe lots of guidance is the right thing in many instances. Maybe not. Where do you and your parents and your siblings stand on this one, and are you involved enough to be there with her when the surgery or anti-depressant is being discussed? It's time to start these discussions about decision-making. Time to begin to ask for more time. Short of a crisis, don't be rushed. It's often okay to have choice play out over weeks, not days.

Evaluate Denial

Thirty years ago, a wise psychiatrist pointed out to me that denial was very helpful for many individuals in the middle of a crisis—as long as the denial wasn't practiced by the circle of family and supporters surrounding the person in crisis. Denial can be both a person's strength for coping and yet a curse at times. Remember that not all resistance is true denial—the immovable position of nonengagement taken unrelentingly over a long period of time despite others' concerns. How do individuals in your family value and use denial? When parents' habits of denial stonewall discussion and prevent thoughtful planning for life's inevitable changes, a family must serve as the quiet anchor in reality. The imbalance between your "power stage" of life and your parents' eroding position of power may simply need more time and gentleness in order to be played out fairly and with trust.

START ACTIVELY PRACTICING YOUR NEW ROLE

Assess Your Parents' Health Habits with a "Seventy-Two-Hour Visit"

Over the course of three full days, just go and be with your parent without escaping into your own preferred activities. This means no Internet, no golf, no gadding about with old friends, no cleaning the apartment from top to bottom. It means being a good guest without nagging, prompting, or commenting. Observe the character of your mother's hours; the personal habits of exercise, nutrition, and hygiene she routinely practices; the social nexus she moves within. This sympathetic, nonjudgmental fact-gathering is a starting point for future conversations about healthful habits.

Not all "slow slip" is irreversible—regardless of your age. Study after study on exercise shows that even elders can regain muscle strength and improve their physical capacities. If your mother has not already incorporated some daily exercise into her schedule, the Station of stability is the time to get at it. Encourage her to get out and walk with friends after dinner instead of turning on the TV. Accompany her while you are there, and observe her relative stamina and balance. Find out if there's a nearby yoga or low-impact exercise class where she might meet other vigorous and supple seniors.

Improving one's diet actually makes a person feel better—it's not all about losing weight. Is she much of a cook? There are lots of well-rounded, inexpensive, ready-made meals to be found in the grocer's freezers. Help her learn to read labels, buy better foods—it's one of the easiest ways to maintain health.

Make sure that your parent is getting appropriate rest. Exercising vigorously might require more rest. Age alone might require napping. Yet taking too many naps can make for difficulty sleeping at night. The "right" rest pattern is highly individual. Help your parent to understand this. Encourage meditation time—praying counts; so does sitting with the TV off and paying attention to immediate things like the birds and the weather. It is never too late for a health and diet makeover, not even at this stage of life.

Admit Your Own Slow Slip

Do you make it comfortable for your parents to admit to decreased capacities by acknowledging your own? Talk to your children. Ask them to describe the changes they perceive happening in you. Ask them what their worries are for you. This may help you frame the discussion you're having with your parents. Plotting out your personal course of change may make you more sensitive to what they are facing. Acknowledging our limits can make us stronger. By the way, it happens that very high-functioning "senior athletes" don't really fall off in their peak performances until age seventy-five, suggesting that sedentary living, not aging, is what "slows us down." Perhaps it's time to model behavior by pulling yourself up another notch. After all, isn't that what you are asking of your parents?

Get to Know the Members of Their Community

By age eighty your parents may be adrift from their community. Many old friends have died or moved away. The neighborhood has changed. Can you identify who is still there to reconnect with? Are your parents partially the cause of their own isolation? Have they stopped going to church or other community events? Have their horizons narrowed to a chair in front of the TV? Changing communities, even more than changing residences, can cause a lot of anxiety and take a lot of energy and still not necessarily get them farther ahead. Wherever they go, they will have to work to establish their identity again. Is it better to invest in what they already have? On the other hand, many individuals who were reluctant to leave the isolation of their old homestead are amazed at how renewed they feel in senior living facilities among the company of others.

Overcome Generational Isolation

Whether parents decide to stay where they are or go someplace new, keep in mind the boost they can get from being around people from various age groups. Can you draw in grandchildren or great-grandchildren for visits once in a while? Facilitate outings or visit concerts, zoos, and museums where there are children and younger people to watch and interact with. At times it is perhaps more tiring for your parents to be around people who have more energy than they do. Your parents may want to leave at the intermission or shut the bedroom door and take a nap before dinner. On the other hand, they may be able to absorb a little of that energy and stimulation and direct it to shoring up their own mental and emotional health.

Put Some Serious Work into Advance Directives

A living will and a durable power of attorney for health care benefit from lengthy discussion. They are not simply legal documents. Go to work on getting your parents to say and then write down how they would like to be treated if they lose the capacity to make their own decisions. (Their responses may be surprisingly different from each other's and your own.) Straightforward talking about these wishes can help the family to better understand and support future decisions. Everyone needs to learn to talk about and be comfortable with the process of decision-making. Practice together in practical areas outside medical care—say, by discussing larger purchases your parents may be contemplating or perhaps travel plans. In the process, identify your family members' various decision-making styles. Ask your family and friends to describe how they have seen one another make decisions in the past—and how it has worked out. It may turn out that "the acorn doesn't fall far from the oak." On the other hand, some family acorns don't end up looking (or acting) like oaks. You may as well get prepared. There are plenty of different advance directive forms available through state governments and aging organizations. Pick some up and share them.

Create Traditions

Has your mom been a faithful committee member or volunteer? Has Dad got a Saturday morning breakfast group? Activities in your home and community that reflect who parents are and what their lives have been about are a means of attracting attention to their continuing role in the family and community—and they give an elder something more to do. Get your children involved—let them record some oral history interviews. The very process of thinking up provocative questions can be a rich opportunity for sharing and participation with your own children, who may have different and very interesting new questions to pose. Ask to hear your parents' stories again, not just the familiar nuggets, but reaching for other memories while their voices are strong and their wits are keen. Later, when talking and remembering are more difficult and spotty, you can give back these salvaged memories, sharing the family's narrative wealth with grandchildren and great-grandchildren. Digging through old photos, making albums, gathering the names and dates, and perhaps even learning media skills or teaming with someone who can make a video or computer slide program can help your parent create a connecting legacy. How about having the grandchildren explore the garage or attic to rediscover what traditions may have been forgotten? Check in with your local historical society. Be more hands-on.

Promote an Ethical Will Project

If either of your parents wants to tackle a bigger and more enduring personal project, introduce them to the writing of an ethical will. This age-old tradition of elders' summarizing in a written statement their experiences, beliefs, values, wisdom, and advice can be a wonderful project to promote. Help your parents get started by conversation, perhaps recorded, that gives them the food for thought to whet their appetite for the actual writing. Take it on as a multiyear project, cheerleading when the writer's spirit flags. This project will keep your relationship filled with conversation topics for years to come.

BUILD YOUR ADVOCACY TEAM

Re-engage the Family

After all those years of people going their own ways, get ready for more contact . . . indeed, much more intimate contact. Society still expects that "family will show up" (so do health care systems when elders are in need). Elders soon learn that having people with them who know them when the going gets tough is of great value. Marshal these loyal forces and get reacquainted. Observation has it that at no time since adolescence are parents and children so entangled.

Generational differences can be matters of style that may obscure an essential harmony of values. But there may also be significant differences of outlook and need. Ask your parent to share the stories going around in "elder spheres." Elders are always talking about their adult children at lunches in senior citizen centers, and adult children are describing their parents to friends at coffee breaks or over dinner. Now is the time to share some of these stories within the family and to compare notes before you actually have to function in a time of crisis.

Anticipate the Onset of Interdependency

"Mama ain't happy, ain't nobody happy." When crises come for frail elders, the ripples spread all around. It pays for everyone in a family (and to some degree for friends and neighbors) to recognize that working to keep problems from getting out of hand, then swelling into a crisis, benefits everyone. After ambulances (or police) have appeared once or twice on the scene, a family will appreciate that everyone is in this together. Don't underestimate the impact of avoidable crises on work time, family plans, and holidays, and your commitments to your school and college-age children. Take a look at what your employer may offer in the way of pretax "elder care" accounts, which are similar to offerings for child care programs you may have used.

If you can get your parents to work in a Slow Medicine partnership with you now, not only will you be helping them, but you will end up avoiding some of the 30 percent of all emergency room visits that are viewed as simply failures resulting from inadequate primary medical care.

ENGAGE MEDICAL CARE
Talk with Busy Physicians

Your elder's physician can be a great resource, but if you are coming from far away and entering into a new medical system, you may not be able to identify your parent's primary physician among a stable of others. Finding a way "in" to a closer working relationship with your parent's doctor requires being savvy, patient, and assertive. Show up at office visits with different combinations of family members, expanding those one-on-one, behind-closed-doors visits that doctors favor. Get to know the office staff. It may not get into the medical record, but visibility is raised by letting the staff know "who cares." Find out the preferred ways to communicate with the office. Ideally, you are all committed to the same goals and for the long run. Be sure to ask if that is likely to be the case. Many doctors are working less frequently now outside the office setting, leaving care outside of routine office visits in the hands of doctors who won't know you or your parent. Find out if that's going to be the case.

Get Acquainted with HIPAA
(Health Insurance Portability and Accountability)

At some point a misinformed or inexperienced (and possibly recently trained) medical care worker will bring up HIPAA and suggest that you are not entitled to medical information about a parent or grandparent. Although it's true that the importance of confidentiality is recognized by all in the medical profession, this is the time to work out expressly with your parents and their doctors your desire to be their advocate. Having done so, you may then, if confronted, point out gently to well-meaning staff members that Congress never intended to keep loving families from being involved with the care of their older members. Elders in Late Life need all the support they can get. That's what you're here for. Be polite and persistent in letting everyone know that you are here for the long run.

YOU MAY BE thinking that all these recommendations really aren't urgent, and you are right—probabilities certainly are in your favor . . . for the short run. Adjusting course with your parents can be quite an undertaking. "Perhaps I'll do it, but I don't have the time right now." An elder can reside in the Station of Stability for years, sometimes for a decade or more. You could take a chance and put things off.

Many families resist early discussions about their roles in the first part of the aging cycle, labeling these discussions with their aging parents as "premature." "My parents remain very capable. I respect their independence and would feel hesitant and perhaps guilty intruding into their lives." "You're suggesting that I will have to deal with my siblings another time, and I don't want to go through that again—growing up with them was hard enough. They're going to let me do all the work anyway." Or, "After the divorce, they went off on their own as far as I'm concerned . . . and their remarriages make it even tougher—all those extra people to deal with."

You may be asking yourself if this approach really has value. You may have your hands full with stability problems in your own relationships. Or your newly found freedom with the children out of the house feels so good. What is in it for you? Where is the pleasure or satisfaction? Can you be guaranteed that this is worth the time, effort, and stress? Perhaps your parents may change their wills if you get "too pushy."

You are right to feel this way; your parents may be hesitant too. But the need for a "relationship agenda" will not go away. If you put your engagement off for now, be sure to come back regularly to review the wisdom of your decision to delay.

"Even bringing up the subject of advance directives makes them nervous," Jane said during our hallway discussion. "They get very suspicious." "Be gentle," our team's nurse practitioner replied. "Let them live with the idea for some weeks or months. But don't *you* forget that it is still important."

Compromise

⸺◦◦◦⸺

"Mom's having a little problem."
—DAD

In February, while the snows were deep and cold in upper Michigan, Bertha, at eighty-six, took her longed-for trip with me to Hawaii. Her limited stamina initially restricted our plans to one major activity a day, but after the third day, we were taking half-mile strolls on Waikiki Beach, riding buses about town, touring the island— Pearl Harbor and Hanauma Bay—in our rental car. On Bertha's return to Michigan, a follow-up visit with her family doctor showed that her blood pressure was up a little, and so a new "water pill" was added to her regimen. She didn't think to tell me about the change. Such a little thing. As spring came on and the days lengthened and became gradually warmer, Bertha felt her balance worsen a little, here and there, but not enough to mention. Stoic and uncomplaining, she'd share that little observation with her doctor if things got worse. Besides, she was looking forward to an early summer visit with the family and didn't want to risk upsetting that plan.

A pivotal hour during that subsequent visit is seared into my memory with regret. The newly introduced "water pill," taken by then for four months, caused her to slowly become dehydrated and to lose dangerous amounts of potassium from her system. She was one of the people for whom this common group of "water pills" also causes upset of delicate insulin and sugar metabolism, turning a mild case of diabetes into its full-blown crisis form. The early summer day started out like so many others. Bertha wanted to return some books to our local village library. A strong and regular walker all her life, she had often covered the half mile into town with ease. Knowing how important mobility is to an elder's well-being and how proud Bertha always was of her daily excursions, my wife didn't insist on driving her. This time, however, the afternoon proved unusually warm. By the time she reappeared at our home, Bertha was literally staggering, so weak she could barely pull herself up the front steps by the rail. She was more flushed and distressed than we had ever seen her.

THERE IS A time, late in a northern winter, when the firm, weight-bearing ice on ponds, lakes, and rivers begins to melt down and "break up." This natural subsidence seldom occurs in a continuous, predictable way. More often the surface warming by day is somewhat offset by cooling at night, giving rise to a covering layer the strength of which is very difficult to assess. Moving currents can carve out channels; shoreline areas generating reflected heat create treacherous spots close to the seeming security of the solid ground of the shore. Hearty souls who venture out to enjoy the ice fishing season and want it to extend its pleasures just a bit longer must consult their past experience to make just the right call about when the risk of falling through becomes too great.

For an elder, the Station of Compromise is about vulnerability in changing circumstances. We sense the passing of a season; at the same time, we long for it to remain. We should not lightly give over this sustaining sense of familiar patterns, habits, and ways of being. And most elders do not . . . even when "the ice is thin and treacherous."

In the landscape of our older family members' lives, there will often come an event that forces a changed awareness of an elder's limits. In time, and with the clarity of hindsight, families may come to regard one little decision or unobtrusive happenstance as a kind of watershed in the life of a loved one and the whole family. No matter how carefully an elder may have been attending to a regimen, slippage comes. "It wasn't like him to do that." "These trips are more challenging than they used to be." "If only we'd realized how hot it was." Often the initial insights aren't verbally reported or shared until change has been certified by a doctor's comment or diagnosis, or by cascading later events that led to a crisis. And even then, full acknowledgment and distribution of information within the family and among friends may remain very limited.

"It's clear to me that these trails up the mountain are getting steeper," Stan admitted to his son during the last hike. That changed awareness for this active seventy-eight-year-old forced a rare visit to his doctor, whose tests uncovered a blood abnormality, a slow-moving leukemia. Although the doctor's recommendation was to "stay in close touch and just follow the numbers" (that is, don't rush to start a treatment), a swaying sword of Damocles now hung over this accomplished outdoorsman—at least in the eyes of his family. "You could fall and bleed to death, or put yourself in circumstances where you'd have a heart attack," they worriedly advised. It took more than a year of demonstrating his physical capacities before the family relaxed and accepted his continuing outdoor life. Nonetheless, the hike before the diagnosis marked a watershed moment for this elder and his family.

At this juncture of an elder's Late-Life journey, the overriding problem for the family is that our understanding is clouded by so much else that is going on in our lives—work, children, our own health, and community commitments. Being helpful to your parents during this "transitional time" requires being quietly and constantly on the lookout for areas of important change in their daily lives. It also requires devoting the energy and patience to diplomatically negotiate your evolving role. The effort required can vary greatly in intensity and duration, depending on the need. Trying to coach Mother to be a more informed and assertive patient when trying to learn about her lab test results means going against her habits of a lifetime. Against these habits of passivity and denial, in distracted circumstances, it takes a conscious effort for everyone involved to evaluate and begin to respond to this changed territory of "softening ice." Those concerned for an elder's well-being must practice patience and positivity while persevering through fogs of sudden uncertainty.

The Station of Compromise for the family is first and foremost a time of vigilance and ready attendance. For however long it lasts—and it may last for years—this station requires the steady application of available energies toward watching, analyzing, interpreting, and communicating, and then learning about and choosing among varieties of medical and/or social resources on an elder's behalf. Diplomatically joining your parents' conversations with their doctors requires tact, time, and belief that you are adding value to the care they are getting. This careful and persistent practice of involvement and vigilance seeks to avert and forestall the imminent crises that threaten to emerge from the pack of six or seven diagnosed ailments that are at work and unfolding in your parents' life. At this juncture in the family's shared practice of Slow Medicine, your goal is to acknowledge and observe the range of issues your parent faces. These issues usually don't require action on your part right at this moment; but they do benefit from all the thinking that goes on subconsciously once you are aware of problems. So many family members have told me that this simple awareness allowed them to sleep better at night.

What Geriatricians Know

In the kind of comprehensive elder care system that I have overseen and managed as the chief geriatrician at Kendal-at-Hanover, the most important community investment directs available care resources toward maintaining residents' capacities to live independently. The goal is to *postpone as long as possible any decline of function* that might require "institutionalization" in the nursing home. Once a resident enters into formal long-term care, the financial burden on the entire system grows dramatically.

Geriatricians, as opposed to disease or organ specialists, are experienced with the many-faceted, multilayered combinations of ailments and disease diagnoses that fatten the charts of their elderly patients. We are keenly aware of the continually changing dynamic among options and the subtle evaluations that are required for the coordination of our patients' multiple therapies. And we are used to working in coordinated teams of caregivers, providing as informed and comprehensive as possible a response to needs while maintaining regular communication with a family. If the issue is coordinating care for cancer, our lead team member might be the doctor; if the issue is restoring mobility after an injury, it would be the physical therapist; for a bout of depression, it could be the social worker.

As a result of our appreciation for the complexities of this special time of life, geriatricians have created systems for describing and grading elements of an elder patient's life situation that are very different from focusing on the statistics of disease states. You may hear your doctor or other medical caregivers referring to your mother's ADLs, IADLs, or AADLs (activities of daily living, intermediate activities of daily living, and advanced activities of daily living). As with all measurements, such evaluations have to be seen in the context of the individual. These particular descriptions pinpoint where compromise begins. In fact, the federal government uses these descriptive categories to determine an elder's eligibility for home support programs or nursing home admission.

The Station of Compromise is a good time to assess all of your parents' activity levels. On the basis of the careful observations you made early on while visiting your parents during the Station of Stability, you are in a good position to judge which activities that previously had been an easy part of their daily routine are now under threat. These judgments will help the whole family evaluate what exactly is being compromised.

Activities that require some planning to accomplish, AADLs are the activities a person needs to be able to do for himself or herself in order to live as an active, participating member of the community:

- participating successfully as a member of a group—quilting bees, choir, volunteer projects
- leaving home to meet social needs—going to church, attending meetings, visiting friends' homes, attending events and performances
- using public transportation, driving a car, traveling
- shopping beyond simple grocery needs
- enjoying an out-of-home exercise routine
- assessing and coordinating home or car maintenance and repair

IADLs are what people need to be able to do to live by themselves in an apartment, having their groceries and other services delivered, and being accompanied on outings. These activities include:

- moving around adequately and safely in the apartment, navigating stairs if need be, possibly going downstairs to collect mail, using an elevator
- making the bed, cleaning up, doing light housekeeping
- simple cooking
- making telephone calls
- keeping track of bills and writing checks

Basic ADLs are what people need to perform by themselves if they were to live independently in a bedroom/bathroom suite in a house with an attentive family nearby. Without ever needing to leave their quarters, they would be able to accomplish their own

- bathing
- dressing
- using the toilet
- moving from the bed to the chair and the chair to the toilet, that is, basic mobility
- eating without help

(These activities are listed in the order in which these basic capacities are usually lost.)

IN MOST STATES, an elder's dependence on others for performing two or three ADLs is enough to qualify for nursing home care. Yet for every person so dependent in a nursing home, studies suggest that there are two other elders just like that person who are being looked after at home by family members. All cope with similar problems—declining mental capacities and chronic debilitating diseases such as heart failure, diabetes, osteoporosis, and chronic lung disease.

The Driving Dilemma

Growing old and progressively frail entails the loss of habitual levels of activity and personal competencies, and, along with them, cherished kinds of autonomy. As an example of work to be done at this early Station of Compromise, I encourage families to begin to talk about driving because it remains of central importance in most elders' lives. Enter into a discussion of this subject unprepared, and you will find yourself challenged (appropriately) by older drivers fiercely protective of their way of life. Losing driving rights in our culture is viewed as a catastrophe because it has such a huge impact on the hope of meeting one's practical needs from day to day . . . not to mention the psychological effect on one's diminished identity in our car-centered world.

But let's look at reality. When I honestly examine my own experience, I know that right after medical school I voluntarily gave up my marathon cross-country driving (fifteen to twenty-four hours straight with rotating drivers); I gave up discretionary bad-weather driving when I had a young family; and for the past decade I have preferred not to drive at night for any distance. Sometime later, as my eyes and span of awareness weaken, I will shorten further my day's driving hours on a long trip and give up all long-distance night driving. Still later, I will forgo driving in Boston and avoid the high school area at the hour school lets out. Then I will scrap all night driving outside my own community, stay off urban expressways, and eventually stay off all interstate highways and shopping mall parking lots. Next, I will drive only to the local grocery store and post office in daylight hours. Finally, I will not drive at all in winter and will drive only between 6:00 and 7:30 P.M. in the spring, summer, and fall when, in my community, traffic is light because most others are at home eating dinner.

In other words, I will repeat in my own life what my older patients have taught me about their stages of giving up driving. Even then, I suspect, I will be reluctant to hand over my license because I "might need it for an emergency." Eventually, the fear of having to take yet another driving exam, including a road test, will lead me to let my license expire. With this plan, I hope my children, or the police, won't ever have to confront me with my own malfeasance. Sharing these considerations within the family is good practice in empathy and understanding.

GERIATRICIANS KNOW THAT careful, repeated analysis of a patient's functional AADL, IADL, and ADL capacities highlights the interplay between the functional measures of an elder's physical, emotional, and psychological health and a family's available resources for physical and social support. The work to extend an elder's stay at the Station of Compromise requires maintaining balanced planning within the family using a Slow Medicine approach. Talk about this over weeks and months; don't simply give an ultimatum. It takes time and careful consideration among all involved to promote everyone's recognition and acceptance of a changed reality. This means talking about uncomfortable things. Take care to emphasize the skills and abilities the elder individual still has. Avoid panicking or prematurely ending his or her independence. It takes time for a parent and supporters to adapt, downshift, and get comfortable with new limitations. At the same time, the family's newly shared awareness of change encourages talk and the kind of practical explorations that can result in increased social support at home. Better planning can make more hands available for day-to-day care and oversight of matters like improved home safety through the use of bathroom bars, walking aids, and better lighting.

Compromise is the station for education and consultation. Learning when to avoid inappropriately aggressive, or premature, approaches to care, gathering conservative options instead, and working out the practical requirements of these decisions with family members are crucial for success. Commit now to a much more measured process for making medical decisions. Don't get swayed by overzealous surgeons or media advertising quick fixes for problems. Given an elder's fraying web of well-being, instituting ill-considered testing, drugs, or medical procedures may pose a greater threat than taking no action at all. Poor sleep, indigestion, incontinence, constipation with soiling, and depression are seldom "fixed" by a drug alone.

Compromised mobility (one of the most sensitive indicators of a person's overall well-being, affecting everything from digestion, circulation, balance, and strength to overall emotional health) might simply be solved by taking your parent regularly to a podiatrist to remedy ingrown nails, ill-fitting shoes, and bunions. Carefully chosen elective surgeries (such as cataract removal or timely joint replacements) can, if elders and their families are properly prepared, improve the quality of life by delaying physical dependencies requiring long-term care.

Two Models of Care

Now is the time for families to acquaint themselves with the practical and philosophical differences between two distinct kinds of care available for seniors. Before our hospital/medical industry became so successful and pervasive, families took care of elders at home. The social model is an extension of the kind of hands-on care a family with many children living nearby, or, quite commonly, a daughter or son in her or his own home might provide. This way of caring does not emphasize the use of professionals and is more akin to the traditional "chair by the fire" approach in which an elder is looked after and kept warm, safe, and close to the center of activities. Perhaps, as I once observed in Italy, Grandfather sits on a chair by the front door of the house on the village square, and one child or another, or a friend or cousin, comes by every little while to walk Grandfather around with him or her doing the daily shopping. In the Caribbean, when Grandmother can no longer look after herself and cannot walk safely alone, she is taken into a daughter's home and given a mattress on the floor to keep her from falling out of bed and breaking a hip. She is bathed and fed each day. Her linen is kept spotlessly clean. The babies play beside her on the floor. Visitors and family members pay their respects when she is not sleeping. She still has her place in the extended family, even as her strength wanes along with her appetite. The social model is hands-on, family-centered, and focused on the fabric of daily care in the home with all its personal touches.

The tremendous power and value of the social model are not well understood by many physicians, yet this model is the bedrock of a family's practice of Slow Medicine. I have seen families that instinctively, and successfully, fall back on an intense application of social and emotional support as a first effort to deal with, for example, newly discovered, unsettling conditions such as memory impairment, depression, or even physical problems such as a new diagnosis of mild angina in a frail parent. Personal support has long been recognized as a way of offsetting new stresses. This is Slow Medicine in its most powerful form.

In fact, the first stage of Slow Medicine is often not drugs or procedures but a mobilization of caring hands—family, friends, neighbors, local and nonprofessional caregivers. Familiar faces help elders maintain their sense of personal identity. Because elders are not relocated to unfamiliar surroundings at the first sign of compromise and new needs, their personalized space, favorite chair, and footrest continue to boost their spirits. Rest is better, and the cat still sleeps reassuringly on the bed. Food preferences and timing of meals are tailored to their lifelong habits. Home is a setting where alternative and complementary medical practices can now be easily introduced—relaxation, therapeutic touch, massage, perhaps new herbal teas, quiet imaging skills. Once the threat of formal medical care is eliminated, elders may be more receptive to these other approaches. Perceiving choice makes new options more palatable.

Now, this very rosy scenario can work only under the best of circumstances. When does the social model break down? Help and support may not be so readily available. They may even "peter out" with time, as stresses mount on those who shoulder the heavier burden. The ultimate fear of caregiver burnout always looms over the social model, especially when the base of support is too limited. This is a very common problem. Financial costs may also increase, since there is little or no insurance coverage by Medicare or Medicaid for these true "health maintenance" activities. There is always the possibility of an elder's needing to be uprooted if further medical approaches are needed (sometimes accompanied by guilt-inducing "I told you so" comments from relatives or professionals). My family had a few naysayers who sniped a bit from the sidelines when a Slow Medicine approach for my mother had to be balanced with medical interventions.

The Social Model in Senior Living Communities

Today, pacesetting senior living communities (SLCs) judiciously seek to coordinate and combine their social and medical programs. Keenly aware of how much added expense must be borne by their communities once a resident requires extended nursing home care, these SLCs are quick to intervene with balanced applications of the social and medical models of care before a situation comes to crisis.

SLC "baseline support" programs offer a homelike setting in independent apartments, assisted living suites, and a nursing home. Social support is readily available from the paid staff as well as, over time, a developing circle of concerned friends. Nutritionists offer varied menus. There are many recreational activities available, and many of these facilities have been planned to encourage walking. The best of these organized communities facilitate continuing exposure to the larger world and mixed generations through on-site child care and elder-care programs. Enlivening arts and learning programs, computer instruction, and shared social events like movie nights and talent shows enrich one's days and keep one's mind off discomfort, pain, isolation, and limitations that might otherwise end up being addressed only in the doctor's office.

In general, the social model focused on family and community still serves most places in the world. In the richer countries of Europe and in Japan, many social services for elders are coordinated and paid for in what is essentially a government-supported brand of Slow Medicine.

The Medical Model

We all recognize the value of good acute medical care delivered in emergency rooms and hospitals. Television, in phenomenally successful shows such as *ER* and *Grey's Anatomy,* touts with pride acute care as it is practiced by our large medical centers. The economy created by our acute medical care industry make lobbyists and policy makers anxious about changing this lucrative and growing orientation.

Indeed, there are many positive features to this approach to care. Many crises for elders do require emergency and inpatient care. Heart and lung diseases, for example, are common in elders and sometimes require quick interventions. And when urgent care is needed, we know we can turn to professionals with high levels of training who attempt to apply measurable standards and protocols. New efforts to create consistency and efficiency and to learn to manage some of these diseases aggressively in older patients are to be applauded. We have the capacity in our hospitals to administer complex (and costly) treatments very quickly. Some of this hospital care is Fast Medicine at its best, as consistent, readily available, and smoothly produced and pleasing as the top-selling latte at Starbucks.

So what's wrong with this high-tech, Fast Medicine approach for elders? The first major concerns for elders admitted to acute care hospitals are the well-documented areas of danger. The elderly acquire more infections in hospital settings; are exposed to treatment protocols designed for younger, more resilient patients; fall more often during hospital stays; and are more likely to be readmitted for complications related to hospital treatment. Large "industrial-scale" environments like hospitals focus on disease and tend to lose sight of the complexity of an older person. Speed is at a premium, and slower-moving, slower-responding elders don't fit well with the pressured environment of fast medical care. Equally important, this Fast Medicine approach to an elder's care has crept—via doctors, drug and technology companies, and the culture that they create—into nursing homes, home care, assisted living, and day care settings. Available resources are snatched from the social support part of the budget to fund more and more prescriptions and procedures, leaving personal care staffs underfunded and underpaid.

The second big problem begins when elders (whose waning strength may have been sapped by undergoing a complicated procedure) are very quickly wheeled (according to time frames for rapid discharge established for young and middle-aged patients) out the hospital door to begin extended months of recovery and healing. American insurance schemes are skewed toward funding sophisticated in-hospital interventions. The financial and practical responsibilities of paying for expensive drugs, daily hands-on care, transportation to and from sites of therapy, hiring in-home therapists when institutional coverage expires, and absorbing the expense of adult children's time taken away from work fall upon the family's shoulders, a heavy chain of difficulty that hospital staffs are only dimly aware of.

Finally, in Fast Medicine settings decision-making is different, particularly where the role of family and caregivers is concerned. In the complicated technological settings of our modern hospitals, families are sometimes viewed as "in the way" and requiring time-consuming explanations, interfering with an individual patient's choices, compelling health professionals to "protect" their patients from family involvement. By contrast, when patients are at home (in a social model of care), doctors are more likely to encourage the family to participate in decision-making.

Modern medicine has complicated the situations of elders' late life by offering better and more technological means of extending the length of human life while not necessarily greatly improving its quality. Often this has meant turning what used to be brief, acute, life-threatening illness into a kind of prolonged decline or attenuated dying. Cancer chemotherapy trials for elders (for which acute care hospitals get well paid) may offer small chance for success, but can double the burden on the elder when side effects of chemotherapy exact their toll. Even in America, and in the shadow of the finest hospitals, it must be remembered that late-life elders who are not saved by the blessing of sudden death inevitably come to a point in their life's decline where disabilities reign and death follows. Elders, who at the middle of the last century saw their lives lengthening for a short stretch from improved medical care, today very often face a prolonged course of dependence and difficulty rather than improved quality of life.

> Her bedroom, a conversion of the old dining room, was next to the kitchen, keeping her closer to the heat and the flow of visitors for her and her daughters, now both in their seventies. She lay on her side, contracted like a comma, and had to be eased over so I could see the plastic tube protruding from her abdomen. It had been three years since she left the hospital with a prognosis of "just a few months" based on her advanced age and her obstructed gallbladder. She had been viewed as unfit for surgery, her lungs being so fragile and her torso so bent from her softened bones and many spine fractures. "She's just drifted out of sight and care," her daughters explained. "There's no way we could move her into the

car. We've just kept waiting for the crisis the surgeon assured us would come." For another two years, I had her on my home visit route, learning a lot more about her life as a teacher and her pedagogy at kitchen table and bedside discussions. Both daughters and mother were more than well prepared to say good-bye.

As medical science and practices advance, prolonging lives that would earlier have come to an end, the medical profession and our society have increasingly come to rely on a medical model for elder care. This resource-devouring Fast Medicine approach—occasioned by increasing numbers of medical specialists and declining numbers of general practitioners and driven by experimental research, escalating medical technologies, and pharmaceutical manufacturers—has overtaken former allowances for preventive and chronic care and created a culture of reliance on acute hospital interventions, now our primary mode of care. As hospitals become more crowded and the site of more and more technological interventions, basic chronic care for older patients has been abandoned in order for hospitals to function more smoothly, efficiently, and profitably. Following the medical model, nursing homes, rehabilitation centers, and assisted living facilities have proliferated to become the main institutional housing for elders and chronically ill patients unable to be supported at home.

The Elephant in the Living Room—Dementia

We live in an age of information and in a highly complicated, technological society that places great importance on mental agility and cognitive capacity. Of all the conditions of Late Life from which we seem to be running scared, a loss of mental capacities seems the most preoccupying. "I couldn't live that way" is a common response to witnessing another's mental decline. Elders themselves, living closer to larger concentrations of aged peers than do their adult children, may have a more sanguine response, however. Immediate recall of the names of people and things has been escaping them for decades. Tunneling eyesight and lost ranges of hearing have reduced their perceptual awareness. Lapses of good judgment and some inappropriate behaviors have begun to creep in. For elders, jokes abound and soften embarrassment. Wearing a name tag at social gatherings is a familiar aid. Though acceptance is now more commonly the coping style of their cohort, a few holdouts still prefer to be in denial. Often, their families prefer denial as well.

Where physical safety is concerned, a family is usually quicker to respond than when an elder has lost social inhibitions or has become verbally offensive. If Granddad suddenly gets lost driving to the hardware store he has frequented for decades, that's cause for concern. If he unfeelingly berates his long-suffering wife in front of the children at Thanksgiving, deference and good manners often look the other way. Fear of admitting these behavioral changes helps no one. There is value in addressing them early in their course so everyone can learn more about what cognition loss is and isn't, what it may mean, and what it doesn't necessarily mean. Fear and its partner, denial, delay the work of reorienting ourselves and our relationships so that we can be useful to our elders and supportive of their caregivers. The stress caused by a problem is always substantially offset by recognition and mutual support.

Keep a careful watch. That's what this late-life station is all about. Observe behavioral changes. Observe repeated lapses in handling new information. Realize that the road of dementia can be a long one, involving possibly decades of slow decline. The earliest stage may last for many years. Be discreet. Elders with progressive cognition loss may not necessarily benefit from a premature or forceful acknowledgment of their condition. Some may. Your understanding of your elder's character and personality must be your guide here. Talk with your siblings.

Equally important, talk with your parent's friends. How are they handling these changes? Be aware that your elder's partner or caregiver may understand what is happening but may be slow both to acknowledge these threatening changes and to openly ask for help. It may be difficult to move from observations of failing memory and strange behaviors to naming and accepting dementia. Denial may actually help a spousal caregiver get by day to day, particularly in the early stages. Adult children, however, are the least likely to benefit from practicing denial.

If your elder parents continue in a long life, there is a high probability that they and your family will face the problems of a frail or diseased brain. The likelihood of dementia or "senility" as a person ages is the Elephant in the Living Room. Try to accept this idea early on as a given for all future work. Use this awareness as a motive for looking for the positive as early and as long as you can. Be aware that although making new memories is compromised, the ability to respond appropriately "from the gut" in making decisions and offering advice may not be lost in some until much later. Recognize also signs of frailty of the brain as a foreshadowing of the physical frailty that comes with later life. The two can be separate but commonly will overlap at some time along the way. According to community surveys, a quarter of elders over eighty-five and half of elders over ninety show some degree of dementia.

Was she headstrong, impatient, cognitively impaired, or a combination of all three? As a consumer she got what she wanted from the system . . . or did she?

Bernice and her doctor talked about her arthritic hip for a long time, exploring ways in which exercise and medication might bring relief. Finally, her pain and frustration got the upper hand, and Bernice pressed to talk with an orthopedic surgeon without informing her family. A consultation was arranged. All seemed to go as expected, until the surgical date proposed by the hospital for her hip replacement didn't seem soon enough to suit her. Disregarding or unaware of the important physical and emotional preparation advised for any elder contemplating elective surgery, Bernice impatiently (and secretly) called another surgeon to see about available surgical dates in his practice. Lo and behold, she secured a much earlier date for the procedure.

Bernice sneaked off for her surgery with a new physician and with no physical or emotional preparation beyond reading through a general list of preadmission instructions. During her postoperative period, what were once noted as tendencies toward anxiety and impatience progressed to utter confusion. Disoriented by the changed environment and exhausted by the surgery, Bernice never fully comprehended what a proper rehabilitation demanded. Week after week, she remained in the nursing home to which she was discharged for rehabilitation. She never got back to walking independently—or living again in her own home.

Every time an elder falls into crisis, it takes an emotional, physical, and financial toll on everyone. This is especially true of crises that might have been averted by timely attention to detail. Falling into crisis wreaks havoc on an elder's confidence, especially the confidence that one can recover enough to go back to the life one prefers. Furthermore, it is very hard, uncertain work for an elder to get through a crisis and back on his or her feet. Be alert and do all you can at the Station of Compromise to anticipate and head off this situation.

Practical Tasks at the Station of Compromise:

Don't be alarmed by the length and detail of my recommendations in this to-do section for the Station of Compromise. I have gone to such lengths because *this is the station at which careful attending and prompt intervention can make the greatest and longest-lasting difference.*

PUT YOURSELF IN THEIR SHOES

Broaden the Game Plan

Corporate advertising and stories coming at us from the media, rumor, and friends prompt all of us to seek drug therapies for our common problems. But medications have multiple consequences. Don't always turn first to pills. Constipation responds best to diet changes, and the same is true for indigestion. Sleep problems need analysis and attention to bad habits (large evening meals, extended TV watching and reading in bed, late-day caffeine, and alcohol use). Depression benefits from a multifaceted approach including exercise, social support, and listening. There often are effective alternatives to medical prescriptions for the human problems associated with aging. Shared transportation, part-time paid companions, and massage for human touch and relaxation may be just the things to relieve an elder's isolation and anxiety. Today, varieties of complementary, alternative, or holistic medicine may be what first spring to mind, but remember that human webs of regular social support have always existed as traditional means of easing the burdens of being old. Is your family willing to engage in this kind of personalized social investment?

Learn Doctors' Specialized Vocabularies for Relevant Diseases

When another diagnosis has been attached to Dad, be sure to ask questions about any new terminology coming your way. Out of courtesy (or fear of being thought ignorant) many people—old and young—hesitate to interrupt a hurried doctor to ask that he or she try to put things in common language that can be understood. *Cranio-, gastro-, neuro-,* and *cardio-* are terms not known to all, especially if you're older. Having a second listener in the room or using a tape recorder can help, but always add that you want to hear it said in "plain English." After years of attempting to practice the clearer communication needed for Slow Medicine, I still find myself using terms that leave a puzzled look on patients' faces.

Recognize the Limitations of Data Cited from Studies of the Middle-Aged

Research studies, including many studies of medications, do not by and large include older individuals, because it is difficult to find suitable older patients to study: they are naturally somewhat reluctant; they require more time to take in and understand new details; they usually have many concurrent conditions and thus are at greater risk for side effects; and they take more medications that may interfere with outcomes. What this lack of suitable studies translates to is ever-increasing controversy within the medical profession over the appropriateness of making recommendations to elders using evidence that may not be applicable to them. For instance, aggressive screening and treatment for prostate cancer and even breast cancer for those over eighty may actually cause more problems than they solve. Early detection of very small cancers of uncertain danger often leads to more testing for confirmation, which imposes risks, discomfort, and costs without clear benefit. A simple physical exam of the breasts or prostate in the office and home testing cards for blood in the stool are perfectly appropriate low-tech alternatives for detection of cancers that would make a difference in health in elders over eighty. You may find it difficult to question the doctor's recommendations, but give it a try. Doctors may be happy that you are aware of a dilemma that they face every day.

Assess Your Parents' "Slow Slips": Physical, Mental, and Emotional Losses

If you haven't been spending time other than on the telephone with an older family member, or if your visits are busy and brief, it might be hard to observe the small losses that start to govern life after eighty. Getting together now for a few days or, better yet, taking a short trip together periodically may bring to light changes and losses of capacity otherwise obscured. Has Dad stopped eating any fresh fruits and vegetables because his dentures hurt or these foods cost too much or take too long to prepare? Has Mom stopped getting dressed? Fear and coping habits of denial may still delay much open discussion of the implications of these kinds of changes, but this baseline knowledge is important for preventing an avoidable crisis.

Be Aware of Pressures from the "Information Society"

Has modern culture added to your parents' confusion? Much of the urgent "buzz" of contemporary culture is commercially induced and offers little of lasting value. Too often for elders it merely creates anxiety and fear. Are Mom and Dad preyed upon by telephone solicitors and scam artists? "Should I change telephone companies? insurance policies? credit card providers?" Our consumer-saturated age bombards us with information on TV, by telephone, in magazines, and in newspapers, especially about all the problems of aging. New "diseases"—for instance, minimal cognitive impairment, restless legs syndrome, and gastroesophageal reflux disease (GERD)—are marketed to promote increased drug use. Under the cover of medical reporting and public education, commercial interests publish incomplete and indiscriminate research and information—accelerated advertising for Fast Medicine. For the elderly, this cataract of data is confusing.

Somewhere between believing that exercising the brain is desirable and accepting that multi-tasking is much more difficult for the old resides the dilemma facing our elders. If an elder is beginning to be less sharp, and possibly more worried, how about turning down the static by providing entertainment other than TV, thereby diverting or eliminating confusing sources of information and substituting instead more physical stimulation and relationship time? Help elders toward shared activities such as card games or reading aloud and direct them away from the overwhelming flow of worry and fear-inducing information coming over the airwaves. Concentrate on an elder individual's established strengths and pleasures. Focus positively on what can be done, not on what is lost. The broad principle to follow is "More activity, not more information."

Keep Track of Differences Between "Cost" and "Value"

Perhaps something new is being offered—a complicated test at the hospital that will "rule out" a possible, but rare, diagnosis. Or a series of $100 physical therapy visits for a chronically painful knee. Or a new antiarthritis medication that would cost $1,500 over a year. Or a naturopath's recommendation for supplements sold in the office—only $600 per year. Or—something a friend recently called me from Florida to inquire about—a remarkable "four-in-one deal" combining screenings for softening of the bones (osteoporosis) and hardening of the arteries— just $129.95. Everybody is selling something. In our pressured and pressuring health care system, driven by anxiety, we are seldom calmly advised to take time to make a thoughtful choice to determine the real usefulness, or value, of recommended care or treatments. In fact, there is usually so little time allowed for discussion or to seek second opinions that we sign on as soon as a recommendation is made. Very often patients are made to feel ashamed for questioning or voicing reservations. Sadly, under present market conditions, our appreciation of real value comes only in retrospect. Keep in mind that most mainstream and alternative providers are in some way benefiting financially from their recommendations, a lurking feature of Fast Medicine.

TAKE CHARGE

Rebuild the Foundations of Health

Regaining and maintaining the foundations of health are the best insurance against future crises. Back at the Station of Stability, when everything was going well, you made a careful assessment of your elder's health habits. At that time there was no immediate motivation for change. Now things are different. Perhaps your mother is faced with rising blood pressure, some swelling of her ankles. Perhaps she is having some dizzy spells or more frequent upset stomachs. Fortunately, you and your mother agree that improving the ways she takes care of herself (diet, rest, exercise, social engagement, reflection, spiritual practice) can help her through this Station of Compromise by slowly and patiently strengthening her constitution. Her doctors would agree, but habitually focus on problems and weaknesses, offering medicines as a first solution. It's their job. Don't refuse to consider their prescriptions, but encourage your mother to work on building her overall strengths. In fact, work along with her. Learn to be her companion and cheerleader. You may find that she either doesn't need the medication or won't need it for long.

As your mother's body weakens bit by bit with age (and a laxness about self-care), these newly identified problems have gotten converted into "diagnoses" and written into her medical record. By the time she is in her mid-eighties, the "problem list" in her medical chart is often lengthy (eight to twelve items wouldn't be uncommon). Even though she may feel reasonably well from day to day, your mother may become a servant to that problem list. It's your job now to itemize, with the help of friends and family, your mother's personal strengths—"can still walk two miles," humor, fortitude, stubbornness, and character all count. Get to work and focus on how to bring back other capacities she may have lost. Our medical care system doesn't focus on this aspect of health, and Medicare doesn't pay for general restorative services. (Try holistic health care practitioners as a way of getting her focused—they often do a better job at finding the positives.)

Respect Your Parents' Autonomy

"Dad has always been so different." So give him a chance to mull over this latest problem and see what he comes up with. The statistical bell curve flattens and widens out a lot with aging. People have become more distinct, physically, physiologically, and, not least, psychologically. Elders become so different from one another by the later part of life that each responds very differently to illness, stress, and disease. Let the search for his way to solve the problem play out for a while. Increasingly, harried, efficiency-driven doctors with little time for reflection just treat diseases; families, on the other hand, relate to highly complex individuals with surprising, sometimes hidden, sources of grit and resilience. Give Dad time and the chance to find his authentic self and personal approach to his changed situation. He may surprise you.

Build Confidence in Relating to Larger Systems of Care and Insurance

New health issues bring different bills and "this-is-not-a-bill" notices from Medicare and other insurers. At the Station of Compromise, you can expect new (and often conflicting) reimbursement codes, unfamiliar abbreviations, lots of numbers, and startlingly high costs, some of which will probably not be covered by insurance. *For people over sixty-five, about 30 percent of all health expenses are paid out-of-pocket.* Copayments mount up, as do new drug costs. Along with promises of breakthroughs with the latest therapies, a family must consider how various options will impact their available resources—financial, emotional, and practical. Are expensive drug remedies using up money that might be better used in providing more and better social support for elders and their caregivers? As compromises mount, it's good to get grounded for the work ahead. Before there is a crisis in the form of new copayments or uncovered costs, everyone in the family should begin to tackle the challenge of understanding complex medical insurance paperwork. Since it is almost inevitable that this issue will involve adult children over time, engaging in this painstaking work makes sense now.

Practice Decision-Making and Working in Interdependent Relationships

What are the opportunities short of a crisis that commonly come along for families to practice together, developing skills and habits for later hard times? More complex dental care, routine cataract surgery, elective joint replacement surgery, and subsequent rehabilitation regimens—perhaps even a colonoscopy—can become the occasions for practice runs of increased involvement. Many of these procedures are introduced by doctors with "Don't worry, we do loads of these" in an understandable effort to reduce everyone's anxiety. In fact, many elders do go through these procedures without any family attention or involvement. But going along for the ride as an adult child can deepen your understanding of your parents and how our medical care system works as well as hone your personal skills in just "being there."

Practice Witnessing Rather Than Intervening

When you are together with your parent at a medical visit, keep in mind the concept of witnessing (that is, intense watching, listening, and feeling—without taking over). Though you may be used to being in charge of the pace and shape of activities in your own home and life, you are not in charge here, not yet anyway. You may have done this kind of holding back when you taught your adolescent children to drive. Now the task is to watch and learn.

Observe how crucial simple and timely attention to the little things can be in maintaining your parents' fragile patterns of well-being. Rashes, itching, areas of skin irritation, and discomfort can be addressed before elders' thinning, fragile skin breaks and bleeds, leaving them vulnerable to injury and infection. Their dentists can find out if sore gums, denture pain, or even latent abscesses are inhibiting chewing and thus interfering with their nutrition. Most of these won't require urgent attention. Time spent together can build strong foundations for future understanding and trust. Later you can bring up your own concerns one at a time and see if your parents will attend to the problems.

Approach Aging Gently, Accept Disease, Challenge Illness

Separate *aging, disease,* and *illness* in your mind and you are well on the way to having health discussions with much more understanding and depth. But beware: the medical profession doesn't always separate these terms very well. *Aging* refers to an inevitable natural process that diminishes the body over time. You can often accurately identify changes of aging by comparing notes with peers. *Diseases* are abnormalities of the body defined by doctors and medical science that have the potential to cause problems over time. *Illness* is best defined as "being sick," with loss of function and not feeling well. Illnesses are usually caused by diseases, although some underlying diseases may be difficult to identify.

Be aware that changes that occur naturally with *aging* are being increasingly identified, perhaps not appropriately, as *diseases* even though these changes don't necessarily result in actual *illnesses.* Each decade the numbers that define blood pressure as abnormally high keep getting pushed lower and lower, now giving roughly 50 percent of all those over eighty the disease label of "hypertension." A few points more and mild elevations of blood sugar go from "age-appropriate" to formal "diabetes." Joints, naturally deteriorating with age and use, acquire somewhere along the line (usually after an X-ray) the status of "osteoarthritis." Age-appropriate mild memory loss slips over the line to "Alzheimer's disease." The examples go on and on. *Accept without undue alarm the fact that your elder will acquire "disease" labels; focus instead on the real threat to health for elders—the breakdown of health and the onset of actual, and often preventable, illnesses.* After any sudden illness runs its course, certainly you should pay attention to treating a clear-cut disease that truly caused the illness. Equally important, get your parent back to work on foundational health habits to strengthen his or her constitution.

Be a Vigilant Caregiver and Learn Your Parents' Reaction Style

What a delicate dance for your parents and for you, knowing how to react just right to changes in how they feel each day. It's more difficult for them because as they have gotten older they are more likely to feel a broader array of body discomforts. What does your mother report to her spouse, her friends, her family, her pharmacist, her doctor? Over time, patient and family alike can fine-tune their awareness by focusing particularly on newly arising feelings or sensations. Let her talk on about her long-standing light-headedness when rising, cold hands and feet, sleepiness after lunch, and tiredness now "compared to when I could go all day long." You want to help her recognize those few new sensations or symptoms that may require a telephone call to her doctor's office to deal with the worry.

Always keep in mind that while the rest of us with more resilience might sit on some sudden new symptoms for a day or so, an elderly person may actually become sick sooner with the same mild symptoms. A change in temperature, feeling a little nauseated, experiencing a loss of appetite, or having a little bout of dizziness can be significant. In my geriatric medical practice, I learned that it is better to be attentive, usually only briefly and over the telephone, to all ten preliminary patient reports of "not feeling well" in order to meet the one situation of consequence. If acute illness is not detected, acknowledged, and attended to quickly, the likelihood of a real setback goes way up. *This is the essential work of caregiver vigilance so crucial to success at the Station of Compromise. Get on top of illness situations quickly; seek help. Hours make a difference.* If you practice vigilance and early detection, evaluation, and quick response to symptoms and illness, your family may succeed in postponing your elders' further decline by protecting their fragile late-life constitution and shepherding their diminishing late-life energies and morale. An untreated early pneumonia or heart attack may put an elder in the hospital, with all its secondary risks, for weeks. Early response and treatment might even allow an elder to stay at home. Get medical help promptly with the onset of worrisome new symptoms.

Observe Patterns of Mental Slippage

We understand the idea of good days and bad when it comes to our joints. It's also the case for our mental functioning. We often keep an informal inventory of how we feel from day to day. Our generation is comfortable with the idea of biorhythms. Decline in cognition (the ability to process new information) can also happen to elders because of transient fatigue, mood shifts, stress, depression, early illness, medications, and loads of other reasons. Is Mom's voice weaker and is she a little more confused on the telephone in the evening? Could the cause be her evening cocktail, or is she just plain tired? Many, if not most, of these day-to-day changes in memory and thinking may seem less threatening when a loved one and caregivers learn when and why they occur.

BUILD YOUR ADVOCACY TEAM

Learn the Names and Earn the Confidence of Elders' Friends and Unofficial Supporters

When my father-in-law was desperately (eventually terminally) ill in an ICU and the family gathered from distant cities, it was the relationships with his friends of many years that helped guide the family in his care. He had formed his advocacy team (without calling it that), and the team members showed up when they were needed. Two of my mother's younger friends stepped in when she needed some in-home help and supervision. Identify in advance the personal supporters your elders have turned to in their daily lives. Cultivate and value these often underappreciated and underutilized relationships.

Develop a Trusting and Reciprocal Relationship with a Physician Friend

Years ago, stories of the personal family physician were common. Usually he was described as a kindly or crusty old gent who looked in on the frail grandmother, or the child too ill to be taken for an office visit. He knew something, if not everything, about the families he served and was always there when the need arose. Over the years, he became, in effect, a family friend. The days of that style of general practitioner are largely gone, and many among the older generation miss his reliable presence.

Today, in our fragmented medical system, it often seems as though the only way to get any informed advice is to have a friend or family member in the medical business. What families are usually seeking are not the most up-to-date technical care options available (something that can be found as easily on the Internet), but rather how to interact with the right part of the system, what questions to ask before undertaking a particular course of action, and, perhaps most of all, a balanced overview of what the family may be facing.

Nowadays, in the absence of enough personal physicians and geriatricians, the role of "physician friend" has broadened to the point where acquaintances who are nurses, nurse practitioners, specialty physicians, and alternative care practitioners can and do serve in these roles. Look around and see who may be available to your family when the need arises. Running a problem by a knowledgeable professional friend can be a great early strategy. And if you happen to get this advice by telephone from another region of the country, you will also get a better idea of how much variation there is in what is "the right thing to do."

Find the Right Doctor and Establish a Covenantal Relationship

The next member of your advocacy team, if you can find one, is a physician actually involved with your elder's care who will agree to be there whenever and wherever your loved one is in need. This doesn't necessarily mean a commitment to being present physically, but it does mean acknowledging that a part of doctoring is making a covenant (that is, a deep and abiding personal commitment) to be the "go-to" doctor when life is getting complex and medical care is being delivered very impersonally. Many doctors take on this role above and beyond the call of duty inside and outside the office. Others would like to, but are burdened and constrained by employment or practice circumstances that preclude this approach. *It is never wrong to ask doctors about their availability to talk with the patient and family even when a problem is outside their area of greatest expertise.* Ask about a doctor's routines for on-call emergency coverage, especially for elderly patients. Ask about his or her willingness to work with the visiting nurse service or in nursing homes when that care is needed. Be considerate and willing to compromise. Everyone is stretched thin these days. If you can find this kind of Slow Medicine doctor to work with you on your elder's advocacy team, you are well on your way to improved care.

Think About Future Mechanisms for Shared Care with Siblings

Although adult children need not have this conversation with an elder parent present as their referee, starting some informal conversations about future needs at this early stage never hurts (all sons-in-law and daughters-in-law included—consider ex-daughters-in-law and girlfriends when the bonds are strong). Gently try to bring out individual differences in perspective and commitment. Be aware that many issues will cause conflicts that won't be immediately resolvable to the benefit of Mother's care. Pay attention to how family members think and argue—you will be dealing with these patterns in times of higher stress.

Sometimes not all adult children in a family can fit into the advocacy team. Get the lines of responsibility and decision-making clarified when you can, and enlist everyone's agreement.

Awaken Grandchildren to What Lies Ahead

Here is something that surprises: older grandchildren, despite their generational detachment from grandparents at this stage of life, may have just the right combination of maturity and insight into the principal players in the family to offer useful and loving advice from the sidelines. Besides, they are used to doing the learning without having to do the doing. Nieces and nephews can also fit into this category of stalwarts on the team.

Initiate Conversations of Appreciation

When members of the advocacy team are showing their commitment by delivering and doing the work, let them know they are appreciated. This includes medical professionals who can be heartened by good feedback. You should know that much of the caregiving that matters for elders doesn't qualify for Medicare payment; it may be coming as a gift of time and concern. Be grateful.

Make Time for More Visits and Phone Calls

The clock has just ticked past eighty years—don't forget that fact. Make the time and establish habits for more contact with your parent now. No better time will ever come. Everything could go awry in the blink of an eye. Start the conversations. Make the telephone call. Write regular notes or postcards. The connection doesn't have to be long—just reliable. Let parents know you care. (Message to elder parents: This reaching out goes both ways. It's okay to enter the lives of your busy adult children. They will be grateful for your sharing. Do the connecting now, and your children will be better prepared to say that they know exactly how you want to be cared for later.)

Record Essential Stories and Memories

If there is no natural scribe or archivist in your family, now is the time to create one. It's time for adult children to join their mother, who may still be making scrapbooks for everyone else. Pulling out these gathered memories will help later when you are sitting next to her wheelchair in the nursing home and the photos and the stories are among the few things she responds to. With each station of this journey, these remembrances will be of added value. This is a difficult position to rotate in many families if there is no initial taker, but keep at it!

ENGAGE MEDICAL CARE

Bring Slow Medicine to the Doctor's Office

By Slow Medicine, I don't mean taking more time in the doctor's office (something most elders are unlikely to get), but absorbing fully what happens in the given minutes and then taking more time later to sort out the doctor's advice. Recent studies to find out what a lone patient walks away with from a just-completed medical office visit reveal very poor recall of complex information. When that lone patient is elderly, very little clear understanding may accompany the patient out of the consultation room. Using a tape recorder may be one way of getting information to share with family and caregivers, but the doctor may find such a device threatening. Having family members or a friend along on the visit improves general understanding and retention. Doctors tend to speak more clearly and explain more thoroughly when more than one person is listening.

Help your mother prepare for office visits by writing down observations about specific problems, itemizing major concerns, and taking that paper with her. Focus on things that matter to you and your mother and don't settle for a quick review of blood pressure and weight and medications. Be forgiving if the doctor doesn't have enough time at that visit. *Leave your list of concerns with the doctor and ask him or her to think about them.* What you want most to promote at this station is her doctor's reflection and support—Slow Medicine essentials—not a lock-step response that simply shunts your mother along a protocol pathway for tests for diseases. In all likelihood, the doctor wants very much to have more time with patients—it's our pressured, time-is-money system of Fast Medicine that is robbing us of time and quality.

Beware of Fragmented Health Care Systems

You won't believe this until you face it, but most health care is delivered in separate "silos" with poor communication between locations. Doctors' office notes don't get to the emergency room. Hospitals and nursing homes don't communicate well about medications. Test reports are misplaced or are available only in the hospital computer, which the nursing home can't access. Patients and families feel catapulted from one site to the next, trailing records behind them. You'll encounter different professional jargon and terminology, different paperwork, different rules, different insurance codes, different providers, different "cultures." Try to find organizations and professionals accustomed to working together: for example, assisted living residences where hospital, home care, and long-term care are formally connected. Even that won't always accomplish perfect coordination, but it may help.

Request Coordinated Care

Geriatricians know that good care for elders requires a team approach. Never hesitate to bring up the question of how and when, exactly, your parent's doctor or doctors or care teams are going to consult with one another, coordinating their thinking, talking, and planning. When the dentist wants to operate on your parent's tooth abscess, be specific: "Here is the number. Will you please call Mother's oncologist and ask for his input, then talk to us about any differences of opinion about recommended courses of action?" Doctors who refuse or fail to communicate create risky situations.

Begin Monitoring Medicines

Many medicines have been prescribed, often by different doctors, for your mother to take each day, morning and evening, or perhaps even more often. "Take before eating breakfast." "Take on an empty stomach." "Take with food." "Take right after eating." Keeping the pills and differing dosages straight is a challenge for everyone. Were the pink pills really discontinued at her last appointment? Wasn't the dosage on the green one reduced? Is she still supposed to take the medication prescribed by a doctor she no longer sees for a condition that has been "cured"? I recommend bagging everything up and taking it to your parent's next appointment to be reviewed for use, change, or discontinuation. Then throw away the expired or unneeded pills. (Sadly, they cannot be legally passed on to someone in need.) Perhaps you have already helped your parent by buying enlarged, color-coded, seven-day, morning and evening pill boxes. Perhaps you are already the one designated to oversee the correct weekly loading of the boxes. "Mom, you already put one in for Tuesday." Mom's eyesight is not what it once was. Her fingers are not as agile. Don't assume that she's done this important work correctly.

Over and above these daily logistical concerns are more general questions that should regularly be asked of your parents and discussed with their doctors. "Do you think this medicine actually makes you feel better?" "My friend Barbara says she's noticed that taking this medication has made her voice weak." In other words, is the medication in question symptom-relieving or possibly symptom-provoking? Is it being taken because when your parents were changing doctors no reevaluation of their daily drug regimen was made? Is a drug being taken because *some studies* (and it might be important to learn the details of these studies—were they, for instance, financed by the drug company that sells the pill?) have shown that there are *some benefits* (you need to learn more about that, too) for *some people*. Statistical, and sometimes faddish, reasons ("I saw it on TV") are very different from your parents' actually confirming that they noticed a difference for good or ill when they started using the drug. Apart from the question of whether any of the research evidence was shown to be relevant for people of your parents' age, trying to clarify what the drug is really doing for them is an important aspect of beginning to understand the puzzle of their medicines.

Twenty to 30 percent of people taking placebos in drug studies usually report feeling better. Mainstream medicine often uses this argument to explain why patients may say they feel better using homeopathic and herbal medicines, but turning the placebo spotlight on the drugs in the scientific formulary is done less readily. Are the risks of stronger drugs worth taking for placebo gains? Work with your parents' doctors to see how they do with selected drugs. Maybe fewer is better.

Accept the Reality of Trial-and-Error Medicine

Geriatricians know that most prescribing directed toward relieving symptoms (as opposed to reducing blood pressure or altering the results on a thyroid test) requires a trial-and-error approach. In order to cut down on side effects it is always good practice to *keep doses to the minimum needed.* Be aware that once drugs get started often everyone forgets that it might be helpful to reduce the dose and see if the desired effect remains. A second area of concern for geriatricians is the common failure to monitor a new drug closely enough to detect possible side effects. Elders are often asked to return for an office visit a long three to six months after starting a new medicine or having a dose changed. For resilient adults in middle age, this lag time might be an acceptable risk to take. For those over age eighty, with their altered and fragile physiology, it is often the recipe for an urgent hospitalization. *Medication-related problems alone account for an estimated 30 percent of hospitalizations for elders.* You need to be on high alert for subtle side effects after any medication is begun or the dosage changed.

Keep a Personal Medical Record and Share It with the Family

Comparing notes with your parents' doctors is a great way of checking your understanding of what is going on. One way to do this is to encourage your parents to keep, or help them with, the writing of a personal medical record. In this journal, they might note what they understand their medical problems to be, how they were instructed to care for those problems, and how they feel they are doing with that approach. (Obviously, this is a great exercise in sharing information, reinforcing intimacy, and practicing conversation.) This personal record keeping has recently become more widely advocated for those with real monitor-the-numbers diseases such as high blood pressure, diabetes, and congestive heart failure. Keep the record simple and legible and share it with the doctor's nurse at the outset of each visit—or ask if you can e-mail a copy of the latest entries to the office for the doctor to review *before* the doctor sees your parent. More and more doctors are using e-mail to communicate with patients. But don't let "e-visits" become a substitute for your parents (and you) sitting down with the doctor regularly.

Get Acquainted with New Doctor Care Models

New types of so-called "subscription" practice (or "boutique" or "concierge" practice) are springing up to fill gaps in our medical system. For an annual, individually paid fee, these practices provide extra physician services such as prevention, counseling, and coordination of care that are not generally covered by Medicare or other insurance programs. Some practices have sliding fee scales to make this kind of nonacute service more affordable. The true Slow Medicine "practice of the future" may well be modeled on the Medicare- and Medicaid-sponsored PACE programs (Program for All-Inclusive Care of the Elderly). These practices for elders are dedicated to care provided in homes and in the community through teams led by physicians and nurse-practitioners. The initial focus when the program was begun twenty years ago was on frail and cognitively impaired elders, but the scope is now enlarging. These programs are very family-centered and represent the practice of Slow Medicine at its best. Locate a program near you (www.npaonline.org).

THE PACE IS quickening, but the payoff for your timely engagement is bigger than ever. Did you find yourself in denial, sharing your parents' reaction: "I've always been so healthy—how could this happen to me?" Your parents may not need to move beyond their denial abruptly—it may be the reason they are getting by—but you need to wrestle with yours soon . . . because there is real work to do. You now need to get into the circle of their life and get them to share their views with you, not always an easy feat. "You're so busy, dear. I think this will be okay without your getting involved." You need to commit the time and energy now to learn enough about their new problems so that you can be a resource to them. You need to learn about the local health care system they are facing. All this may even require that you prepare for some degree of conflict with your parents and their medical advisers as you struggle to understand what they face. "I know what Dr. Jones is saying, but can we all take a little more time to learn and think about the test result?" This engagement can make you uncomfortable. What is your role? How hard should or can you push against your parents' resistance? Frustration and anxiety may build as you meet the health system head-on. Are you going to be able to compromise your strong views and your own resistance to seeking support from your friends?

Have faith. This is the time to invest "up front"—time is on your side. Trust that there is much value in warding off a crisis through your vigilance and more persistent efforts to nudge your way into your parents' lives. This is beginning to take a little toll on you, but remember that you are still in the foothills on the journey up the mountain. This is training for the heavy lifting to come.

Crisis

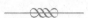

"I can't believe she's in the hospital."
—SISTER

A few weeks after returning home from her summer visit with us, Bertha was back in her own apartment and had just finished bathing, still sitting in shallow bathwater, when she realized that her legs wouldn't work. Even gripping the support bars that had been installed above the tub for safety, she wasn't able to stand. And she wasn't able to reach the Lifeline that hung, tantalizingly, beside the toilet. For a long time, as the water cooled, Bertha wondered what to do. It was late. She had been watching a basketball game on TV. She certainly didn't want to call for help and be found naked by her neighbors. Beginning to shiver, she let the water out of the tub and tried to raise herself over the side by just her arms alone. No go. Getting increasingly cold and desperate, after many tries, Bertha finally managed to hoist herself awkwardly over the side of the tub far enough to grab onto the base of the toilet. Pulling and hauling, wrenching and bruising, she finally managed to slither and bump like a seal onto the bath mat on the floor. There she rested for a while, still unable to stand or reach the useless Lifeline. Finally, after exhausting efforts, dragging herself on the floor by her arms like a commando, Bertha made it to her bedroom. The next morning the apartment supervisor found her scraped, bruised, and in pain when she failed to put out her "I'm okay" sign on the doorknob.

I was distressed to learn that evaluation in the local hospital turned up new rib and spine fractures, uncontrolled diabetes, and dangerously low potassium, the cause of her leg muscles' loss of strength. After two days' bed rest in the hospital, on top of all the other difficulties, Bertha suffered a clot to the lung. This tale is a classic presentation of "first crisis" in the life of an elder.

At this tipping point of first crisis, I encourage families to jump immediately into action. At the early Station of Compromise, you learned to practice vigilance and developed an attitude of readiness. Now those days of static serenity are over: the Station of Crisis takes the trajectory of a short, sudden, and largely unforeseen fall into dangerous water. You may be hundreds of miles away. This is not what you wanted to happen. But you must let go of all the "why's" and "what if's" and focus on "what now?" Understand that despite all your vigilance and careful efforts, some crises will be unavoidable. Suddenly, your parent and you are in well over your heads. Will your parent make it back to the relative calm of the Station of Compromise or sink to a later station from which it is harder to find the way back? Now is the time to think DAMAGE CONTROL.

In my clinical experience, the Station of Crisis is commonly characterized by five elements that families should be prepared for. First, some acute change sets the whole current running, and before you know it you're all caught in a cascade of events, holding on to one another for dear life in very unfamiliar and very scary circumstances. Let's take the elements one by one so that you can understand the experience from your parents' point of view.

1. An acute change in health or circumstances: Call it "thinning ice" or the "awful sword of Damocles," this feared arrival has been waiting for its moment all along. Although it's what you have been working so hard to forestall, it happens anyway. Acute change can arrive in many forms. It may result from the onset of a sudden unexpected illness (bad cold, flu, pneumonia); a sudden accident (a fall or auto accident); a chronic disease running out of control (diabetes needing more insulin to manage or the onset of difficulty breathing because of worsening congestive heart failure or emphysema). Or perhaps an elder has arrived at the limits of tolerance (that is, the elder has run out of resilience and can handle no more stress in the current living arrangement). Perhaps it's really a matter of caregiver burnout, a family's or friends' anxieties overwhelming the situation. Or it's the discovery of a new health issue, a breast lump or blood in the urine. Or perhaps it's an elder's despairing response to being shunted to an unfamiliar location or doctor. There are countless possibilities, and each provokes its own special kind of urgency and worry.

2. The ride to the hospital: Be aware that even beyond the initiating health crisis, an additional crisis may loom in the very choice (or nonchoice) of transport for care. Will your mother be delivered in an unrushed manner to her doctor's office (or the local hospital emergency room) by calm-talking family members? The default position for many elders, and particularly for those who live alone, is a call to 911 made by the frightened neighbor who found your mother ill or in need. Will the ambulance actually go to the hospital where your mother's doctor has privileges? Or will the medics take her to the nearest emergency room? Do you know the names, addresses, and telephone numbers of these hospitals?

Imagine how upsetting this sort of intervention can be. Your mother's private health status has become an object of speculation and rubbernecking in the halls of her apartment house. Suddenly she has strangers coming through the door in unfamiliar uniforms. Then they are down at her side, measuring her quickly elevating pulse, strapping on a blood pressure cuff, putting in an intravenous line, and searching for her medications. Did her attendants find the list of drugs and family telephone numbers posted on the refrigerator door? Things are happening that aren't necessarily being explained. She's frightened now and experiencing a loss of dignity and self-control. Where are these people taking her? What will happen next? Perhaps the EMTs are trying to put an oxygen mask over her nose and mouth. Perhaps they are strapping her onto a stretcher to carry her to the street.

However short or long the ambulance ride is (from rural areas it might be a long one), it is fraught with its own terrors—flashing lights, the whine of the siren, the rush through traffic, the psychedelic array of swaying tubes, the glint of mysterious equipment lurching at every stop. If by some chance you happen to be there, climb in and hold your parent's hand through this experience. Speak calmly. Act calmly. Your very presence will be reassuring.

3. Passing through the emergency room: Years ago you may have spent a few hours in an emergency room waiting for your son to get his broken arm X-rayed and set. Perhaps since then you have been a regular watcher of *ER* on television and think you've become pretty savvy about the kinds of goings-on you may expect there: the handsome Hollywood staff, the dramatic response to emergency arrivals, the climactic heroic measures that have been coherently explained by sage physicians in their wood-paneled offices. Watching such carefully orchestrated, antiseptic action on a flat-screen TV bears little resemblance to the chaotic experience of accompanying your loved ones into that foreign territory as their sole spokesperson and advocate. You probably don't know the protocols or the lingo. You may even find yourself shunted out of the picture completely, caught at the admissions desk filling out paperwork. Family members characteristically get separated from one another—at the very moment when they most need to be together.

One of the first and foremost difficulties of this new situation is the sudden loss of identity that your parent and you will have just undergone. The members of the ER staff have never seen your parent before. They won't know your parent's name or situation or history beyond the brief presenting vital signs and scribbled notes that the ambulance team has recorded. Busy attendants may have no recognition of who you are or what your connection to your parent is or why you are in their way. In many communities, a trip to the ER (even if it has been ordered by a doctor after a telephone or office consultation) means an abrupt disconnection from usual care. The haste of a crisis situation often results in a problem of inadequate information from the medical record at your parent's doctor's office. Your parent's new attendants can't see the present situation in the context of the overall medical history. Even worse, crises often happen at night and on weekends, when the doctor's office is closed and the designated doctor on call is unfamiliar with your parent's situation.

Unless your family has been keeping its own records of your elders' health status along with notes on daily medications and dosages, there is no way under such short notice for the staff to know your parent's real AADL, IADL, or ADL functional levels; the full list of medical problems; or the usual cognitive status. As a consequence of these failures and omissions, in the hurried, pressurized atmosphere of a busy hospital ER, your parent is likely to be the victim of a kind of weary ageism by a staff that seldom has adequate time to get to know its charges. In your parent's anonymity, he or she is in danger of being subjected to rigid, age-insensitive protocols or lost amid the large volume of much more debilitated older patients transferred from nursing homes.

Worst of all, there is a very high likelihood that you are far away and your parent is there all by himself or herself.

4. In the hospital: A hospital is a world unto itself, more like a giant high-tech beehive than anything that resembles your mother's quiet apartment with violets on the windowsill and smiling family photos on the dressing table. Even after you escape the urgency of the emergency room and have taken the elevator up to the appropriate floor, expect extreme busyness: people in various forms of baggy dress moving in and out of the hospital room with a hurried nod and swish, lots more paperwork, and repetitious questions asked by different people as if no one has referred to a chart or talked sufficiently with the previous shift.

Your mother may be exhausted and needing rest, but there are needles and tubes to be inserted, unfamiliar machines emitting beeps on every side, a tangle of thick black electrical cords beside and below the bed, and strangers asking disturbing new questions. "What about her advance directives and do not resuscitate (DNR) status?" You thought the advance directives were on file with her doctor. No one mentioned that this episode was potentially *fatal*. Isn't this an awkward time for such discussions? "Where is her doctor?" "Has the doctor been called?" At first, conversations are very limited and largely unclarifying. Your mother's doctor will probably not have shown up yet and won't arrive until his or her appointment day is over, some hours away, or perhaps not until tomorrow. Or perhaps not at all—if the doctor has arranged for the "hospitalist" doctor to care for your parent. Throughout all of this flurry and hurrying your parent hasn't recognized a single familiar face.

Chaos does not inspire confidence, even though it is typical of these situations. There's tremendous tension at this time of crisis between your parent's need for support and rest and the medical staff's and institution's need for more information. No one has the big picture yet. Individually, the staff may not even know your parent's presenting problem. Everything is done on the hospital's schedule. Noise. Light. Confusion. Roommates. Is it okay to get out of bed to go to the bathroom? Is your parent able to go without help? Is she allowed to? How about a drink of water? Another blanket? Some ice? Your parent is not completely addled, and not a child. Why are the nurses talking with that false and patronizing cheeriness?

For the adult child there are other difficulties. Suddenly, and despite all you know about his remarkable and abiding capabilities, you have to watch your father being treated like a dependent child. You realize with a sudden pang that no one knows your father's history: The extraordinary person he is. The work he has done. His goodness. His fiber. Nor, under these circumstances, is the staff likely to gain such an appreciation. There's too much to do and not enough time. Shifts change too often. You have to start all over with each new face.

Time in a hospital passes slowly for those who don't work there. It's boring to wait in such sterile and uncomfortable surroundings, and it's hard to feel so useless, particularly since you are so used to calling the shots at work or at home. The modern hospital staff trumps the empowered, wise, and prominent "mature adult" you are in the world outside the hospital. Not only is your parent reduced to dependency; so are you. As you watch all the comings and goings, the tremendous cross-hatching of purposes and chores, the complexity and layers of input and responsibility, you will inevitably feel some restlessness to get something done. Meanwhile, the regular hospital staff working around you—administrators, doctors, residents, interns, registered nurses, licensed practical nurses, nursing aides, cleaning and support staff—will all be socializing and casually carrying out their routines. (Can they possibly be paying proper attention to that new bag of whatever it is they are hanging?) All of this will leave you feeling vulnerable and uninitiated.

Although all hospitalizations, of course, will be different and have their own trajectories, in most instances a hospitalization will be of short duration. Average lengths of stay for common problems for elders are often less than one week. There are some typical patterns on the day-by-day hospital journey to watch for. Within twenty-four hours things will most likely have settled down. Much of the rush of evaluations, consultations, testing, and the initiation of therapy will have passed. By the second day your parent should be tired but resting more quietly. You will be able to get some fresh air and take a walk or run an errand, handing over the bedside chair to another supporter.

On the third day, you will be back in place, wondering what happens from here on in. Although you will still be riding the bumps of the trip through the ER and into the hospital, you will have learned the importance of being there as an advocate for and protector of your parent. The first thing you'll notice as your parent comes around from a long rest is that his or her thinking is a lot less clear. Your parent may fade in and out during conversations, dropping off again to sleep.

Confusion and disorientation frequently appear during an elder's hospitalization. The fragile functioning of an older brain, stressed by hospitalization (an illness, demanding treatments, medications with side effects, sleep deprivation, unfamiliar surroundings), is at high risk for "the perfect storm" of delirium, a condition estimated to affect perhaps half of all of those over eighty during a hospital stay. Delirium's "veil of fog" in its mildest form brings on detachment, confusion, waxing and waning of awareness, and some disorientation. In a more advanced form, its effects include rising pulse, dropping blood pressure, fever, and worse. A long list of medical complications (such as low blood oxygen levels, stressed kidneys, mild heart failure, and adverse drug interactions) can contribute to this condition and should be tested for. But, for you, your parent's advocate, the concern is to recognize and report to the nursing staff what you see happening; you know your parent's baseline mental capacities better than the new attendants. If Mother is not herself, take notes and keep emphasizing the changes. She may be able to talk and appear to be conscious and independent-thinking at times, but will she remember the discussions and decisions being made? Probably not. Be aware that in the hospital the diagnosis of delirium is often missed, dismissed as normally what happens to elders when hospitalized. But it can forewarn you of a bigger storm brewing.

5. *Leaving the hospital:* By the fourth day you should start thinking about getting your parent's landing place established—wherever that may be—and it may not in fact be home, depending on his or her condition. If you are lucky, you have thought about this before someone actually suggests that discharge will be in a couple of days.

Be aware that hospitals see their role as initiators of therapy and providers of special technical services, not as places for completing recovery. "There is very little more we [the hospital] can provide that couldn't be provided at home or in a rehabilitation program," the staff will emphasize. Hospitals are allowed a specific allotment of days and a fixed Medicare insurance payment according to a patient's diagnosis. This is exactly where what's best for an individual may conflict with statistically generalized projections. Before the social worker, head nurse, or attending physician tells you that the "only way" the hospital can keep your parent any longer (despite the unsettled delirium) is for you either to attempt an appeal to the Medicare program for an exemption or to personally guarantee a $2,000-per-day payment for "uncovered services," you should ask for suggestions about posthospital services. Remember, the hospital discharge planner wants your parent to have an *average* length of stay for his or her problem, thus saving the hospital from having to absorb the extra costs of longer stays. Now is the time to start thinking ahead.

At the same time, don't waste all of your time and energy on mounting a defense in the hospital. It is much better to have a civil meeting with the discharge staff (this is not a personal issue; it is their job) and then get on the telephone and out and about in your car to explore in person visiting nurse services and nursing facilities. Just show up; you don't need an appointment. You might be assigned one too distant to be useful if you merely telephone and ask. Share this responsibility with other family members. As much as possible, do this work in person so that your family establishes relationships and can call back later in case first efforts fail. Be aware that there will be a lot of additional paperwork. The smells and sights within rehabilitation centers and nursing homes can be discouraging when first encountered. Wheelchairs (with elders in various stages of decline) may line the hallways. Smells in the hospital are antiseptic; smells of rehabilitation are more human. Remember: *this is an early exploratory visit. In all likelihood you are not choosing a final home for your parent at this time* (although that thought may now be flashing through your mind).

The Nonemergency Hospital Admission

Your father's orthopedic surgeon has stressed repeatedly that scheduled knee replacements are "simply routine." He has prepared your father for the hospitalization in a very orderly fashion with a professionally done video presentation, preliminary testing, a carefully timed arrival at the hospital, and staff members who pleasantly usher him along from station to station, task to task. Your father is lulled into thinking, "It's not unlike my cataract surgery." The comforting confidence with which routine hospital admissions are undertaken is in dramatic contrast to the "ride down the rapids" of an unexpected acute crisis. Planned admissions are certainly preferable for the patient and the family alike. Some families may wonder whether they even need to show up given all these reassurances.

No matter what the procedure, hospitals are full of dangerous currents and swirling backwaters that may carry your frail parent into unknown territory. And while it is important to strike a balance between family concern and involvement and your elder's confidence that this is "simply routine," it is good practice for you even in these "routine" situations to be involved and to forestall possible misfortune. Every hospital contact is a learning experience for the family. From the moment your father enters the operating room, the possibility of unforeseen factors altering his course grows. Difficulty with the anesthetic, a burst of irregular heart rhythm, a breathing problem related to some age-acquired asthma or emphysema (previously undetected)—any of these could shunt him into the ICU after the surgeon's success with his "routine" surgical procedure. Be watchful for medication errors or a frail elder's accelerating confusion in unfamiliar surroundings. Being on standby alert and preparing for a more complicated hospital course are your job. You get to absorb the stress of uncertainty while he benefits from the confident preparation he has been given.

The Escalating Crisis at Home

"I know the situation is difficult: your mother is burning out, and your father needs more support—we could see it coming," their physician agreed over the telephone. "However, that is not sufficient reason for the hospital to admit him. I'm truly sorry, but I don't control the regulations." Here you are, facing a characteristic Fast Medicine predicament: responsibility for managing this crisis is handed back to the family. What do you do? Neither of your parents is physically or emotionally ready to apply for nursing home placement and, in any case, that decision takes weeks or months to prepare for properly. Usually, adult children cobble together a plan. "Perhaps Jane can drive over to do a shift with Dad tonight, and then I could get away and be there by tomorrow. We'll have to play it by ear after that."

Patching over problems when decisions can't be made or are too momentous to be made quickly is very common for families of elders with dementia or progressive physical frailty. A chronic problem is not considered acute enough to qualify for transfer to a hospital. Escalating problems with a parent's wandering at night or the fact of no longer being able to move about safely in the home don't meet guidelines for hospital admission or even for medical attention. You may also have learned from past experience that this small crisis may merely be temporary, no matter how mountingly stressful it is for caregivers. Another fruitless visit for evaluation in a busy emergency room doesn't offer much of value. Families must grit their teeth and carry on—or radically change life as their parents have known it.

Recurrent Medical Crises

In your mind, the pattern has become predictable. This is your mother's fourth hospitalization for yet another small stroke. The drill of routine tests and a very short observation period on the Neurology Unit unfold without complication, and she is (almost) back to where she was before this last episode occurred. Living in her own home will always certainly be her preference, but is there any way to stop this in-and-out-of-the-hospital roller-coaster ride? Do we simply wait for the Big One (she has said she wouldn't mind if that happened at her age)? Would she be more secure in that new assisted living place just a few miles from her home? How and when are we going to make the decision?

The Slow Medicine Review

When the scare has passed and you have rested and regained your sense of humor, this is a good time for everyone to take stock in order to *prepare for inevitable future crises*. Nagging feelings of inadequacy plague adult children thrust suddenly into advocacy roles for their parents and coping with the mysterious and powerful institutional challenges of our medical care system. Use this moment of calm to encourage involved family members to meditate privately, then discuss openly, their experiences during the recent crisis.

— What did you fail to understand?

— Were there times when you felt inadequate (emotionally, spiritually, mentally, physically)?

    — Did you in your anxiety blame instead of looking for solutions?

    — At what points did you lack the skills or the vocabulary to do what was required?

    — What skills were lacking? How might you learn them?

— Did you have insufficient support—from family, friends, work, your parent's community, the doctors, and the hospital staff? Could that lack be righted? Do you need to learn to ask for help?

— In thinking back to the chaos of the "trip through the rapids" of the crisis, what did you not get to address with your parent's medical care providers?

— Have you thanked the hospital crisis team? A note or letter to the hospital and staff means a lot to them and lets them know you care and are aware of their good efforts. After all, you may well need them again. (It also will be easier to bring up constructive feedback from a position of mutual appreciation.)

— Has your family formally recruited your advocacy team? Your "physician friend"? This is an opportune moment because of your proven success in dealing with a crisis and your recent emotional involvement.

— Have you communicated properly with your "home base"? Let employers, colleagues, neighbors, and friends know what happened and that you appreciate their patience and support? Alerted them to the possibility that this will happen again? You will be surprised at how many shared stories from their families will emerge.

— Have you set aside space and time to deal with your own emotional needs and fatigue? You are now in recovery too.

— What important words did you forget to share with your parent? your siblings? your spouse? It is always the right time to say "thank you" and "I love you."

So effective was his wife's cover-up that the family was only beginning to get a sense that he was "slipping a bit." Then the eighty-seven-year-old stumbled, hit his head, and ended up in the hospital, where an MRI (magnetic resonance imaging) showed that a blood clot had formed and was putting pressure on his brain. The clot was promptly removed, much to the relief of all.

The "incidental finding" on the MRI was an enlargement of Dad's pituitary gland—"a likely tumor," the doctors said. During a brief consultation with surgeons, the family asked how this discovered condition might have been affecting their father's well-being and how dangerous it might prove, but they received no clear answer. Still, how could they just leave it there once it was discovered? Unaware of the importance of slowing down the process of decision-making and of having his mental status evaluated, the family agreed to surgery, followed by a course of radiation. No one realized how stressful the treatment would be for his fragile brain. That was their father's turning point. Individual family members later recognized their mistaken decision, although it took months to talk about it. Shortly after the surgery, Dad was admitted to a nursing home, his accelerating dementia having advanced to the point where his loyal wife could no longer care for him at home.

Practical Tasks at the Station of Crisis:

GET IN THE GAME

Know What Kinds of Alarm Systems Are in Place in Your Parent's Home

Is there an emergency cord to pull in the bedroom? the bathroom? Who answers that call? Is there someone who checks in on your parent daily? Does this person have your telephone number? Does he or she have your parent's doctor's number? Are emergency numbers programmed into your parent's telephone? Is it time to be looking into Lifeline? Has anyone yet prepared an emergency information package (stored in your parent's refrigerator in a ziplock bag for safekeeping and ready access) that itemizes current medications and dosages, diagnoses, advance directives, and emergency contact numbers? If the ambulance team doesn't request this package, be sure to give it to the team or take it with you to the emergency room.

Learn About the Ambulance Ride

Find out what happens when some well-meaning person calls 911 in your parent's area. Which ambulance services are available? What hospitals do they serve? What is the average response time? What are their protocols for reviving unconscious patients? How much do their services cost? Are they covered by your parent's insurance?

Communicate and Coordinate with the Emergency Room

Too many little white-haired ladies arrive in the ER with no medical record other than the vital signs taken by the ambulance crew and a few scribbled notes taken over the telephone or stuffed into an envelope to explain the problem. Get in the loop as soon as you can. Be sure to get your family's informed overview to the ER staff by telephone or fax. Call your parent's doctor if the doctor hasn't first called you.

Check to see that someone from the doctor's office has faxed over to the ER your parent's most recent list of problems and ailments and what medications (and dosages) your parent takes daily. Ask the ER nurse to let you to talk to your parent on the telephone—your voice can be very comforting in confusing circumstances. If you live farther away, book your ticket immediately and get to your parent's bedside as soon as possible.

Appreciate Hospital Culture

Look around as soon as you enter the hospital. There are "outsiders" in civilian dress, and "insiders" in uniforms. Learn the "white coat" and nursing hierarchies. Take notes to share with other family members. It's been pointed out that hospitals rank right up there with correctional institutions as places where two distinct populations exist side by side, but far apart. Work on being a "bridge." Everyone in this situation is human, but sometimes the connections don't occur naturally. Above all, don't deepen the divide and get labeled a troublemaker.

Get the Story Right

There is an unspoken advantage to specialist medicine: those higher up in the doctors' hierarchy can look brilliant because, by the time they get to respond to the patient's history, the process of winnowing out vagaries that surround any developing illness has taken place. Over time, disparate bits of information have been shaped and focused to help the doctor, the patient, and the family to understand the medical history. Inevitably your parent will edit the narrative of his or her illness at each retelling. Be aware that it's your job to make sure that any "irregularities"—details that are not easily explained by a gathering diagnosis—are not lost. Is the hospital staff hearing that your parent started to "weaken" two months ago? Did your parent's fall last week trigger this crisis? How about the medication change last month? Take notes from the start. *Help your parent to stick with what really happened.*

The hard-to-fit-in pieces need to be reconciled. Often they are the very matters that lead to a better understanding, perhaps even to finding rarer conditions. Keep asking the doctor if there are any loose ends he or she is still struggling to account for. Getting the real story addressed now may save a repeat hospitalization later.

Understand Informed Consent

If you have ever been hospitalized, you will remember how hard it is to absorb the content of all the fine-print hospital forms and releases you sign when you are admitted. Your mind is laced with anxiety induced by stories of other colonoscopies, the confusion and urgency surrounding your sister's Caesarean section, the delays before your son's appendectomy. Fast-forward now to your parent, ill and in crisis, away from home. How much of what is going on can your parent really understand? Even though he or she may be mentally "competent" by medical standards, it is perfectly appropriate to ask that you be involved now as intermediary. Simply voicing your concern raises the level of informing likely to go on. Begin politely to practice your advocacy work here and now right at the bedside. Slow Medicine means that everyone who cares needs to be heard and engaged.

Look Back and Look Ahead

Without pointing a finger of blame, engage your parent's doctor and caretakers in a conversation looking for root causes when things have gone wrong. Know that illnesses present in different, more subtle ways for an elder. Now is a good time to learn from your parent's doctor his or her insights about how your parent's various problems might present as a crisis. Many acute events leading to hospitalization are inevitable, but perhaps as many as half might be avoided. The key here is an attitude of analysis, not indictment.

Listen to and Attend to Other Families in Crisis

"Curiosity dispels fear." A good way to manage your own anxiety and at the same time get a perspective on your parent's situation is by attending to the plights of others—within your family and without. Inquire about how other patients' families are coping. Hang out in the family and visitors' lounge and hear some other stories. Share a cup of coffee. Comfort someone else. Build some solidarity. The nursing staff will appreciate what you are doing. Even three (intense) days around the same hospital ward can create important bonding and support.

Get to Know the Names of the Hospital Staff

Now is a good time to buy a notebook for keeping important names handy. You will need to make notes for absent family members. Good manners smooth human interaction and promote reciprocity. Friendly social exchange between your family and the staff creates a context of caring for your loved one. Introduce family members and friends to the various hospital caregivers who rotate onto the floor and into and out of your parent's room. Personalizing the atmosphere helps your parent to be addressed and treated like the important individual he or she is and warms your own reception when you have to ask for more information or a favor. If there is an erasable board in the room to write on, list all the physician and staff names that your parent and you would like to remember. Keep the list current, shift to shift and day to day.

Protect the Patient

Make sure the nursing staff knows that you are there to help protect your parent from the many unintended things that can go wrong in the hospital and that you want to team with staff members to achieve what should be a shared goal. You know your mother, how well she has been, what her usual capacities are, and how ill and vulnerable she is at this moment. Keep her oriented in strange surroundings by identifying places, persons, and even the day and hour if need be. Offer your input to balance the timing of her friends' visits and to protect her rest and routines. Avail yourself of new Internet technologies (www.thestatus .com, www.CarePages.com) that simplify the process of informing others about your parent's condition and save your having to repeat the same information over and over. Protecting your energies is important too.

Prevent More Harm

Much more is coming to light in medical literature and media accounts about errors made during hospitalizations. Patients are being given the wrong drugs, wrong doses, wrong procedures. While a hospitalized middle-aged person can barely maintain some sense of what is going on about him or her, an elderly person has only a remote chance of understanding what is happening. Most geriatric doctors I know would not want their own parent in a hospital without a family member in attendance *at all times*. (Granted, this is not always possible, but it is still the gold standard of care.) Make gentle inquiries about every test and every drug that is being administrated. Check the labels. Ask if a list of your parent's medications could be left in the room so that you are better able to ask questions about their use. Someone in the family will need to be learning about this by the time of discharge, so it is never too early to begin.

Push Back Against the System

Precipitating a battle around the care of your parent seldom helps; similarly, being completely passive will not serve your parent well either. Try to find out about specific goals that the doctors and staff are trying to achieve (including the goal of discharging your parent as quickly as is appropriate). Speak up. Clarify your goals as they emerge so your family and the hospital staff remain on the same page. Work with your family and various caregivers to come up with suitable options. ("Perhaps a day without stressful tests would give her better rest and make her stronger.") Try to come to mutual agreement on what criteria will determine when your parent is well enough to be discharged. One of the most overlooked tests is "Let's take a stroll down the hall together." Observe your parent's balance, strength, speed, concentration, and ability to talk while walking. When does the gas run out? After you have taken your mother on a test run, dare to suggest that the doctor spend a few minutes strolling with her.

Don't Become "the Problem"

Commonly, busy and overburdened hospital staff will want to show patients and their families the door sooner than is appropriate. Don't let your own actions twist the focus of the discharge from your parent to you. Since the conventional wisdom in medical circles is that "difficult families create difficult patients," relocation is one of the regular means of dealing with conflicting views. "We think she (and you) should be moved to the care of Dr. Jones's team of specialists."

Seek Help for Coping in Stressful Situations

Even doctors-in-training require a long time to learn how to deal with the stress of acute crises. You or someone in your family is likely to have a meltdown in times of crisis or accumulating tension. Seek help early when the signs appear. Call in less stressed reserves. Members of the hospital chaplaincy can often help. If someone is reluctant to seek help, go yourself. "Could you suggest how I can help my brother?"

The Healing Power of Touch

Sights, sounds, and smells in the hospital may be disorienting, but the immediacy of touch is calming. Sit close to the bedside. Reach out a hand. Keep it there. Touch is orienting when other senses may be failing. During periods when an elder is delirious or is passing in and out of sleep, keep people in the family or Circle of Concern rotating through that bedside position. So much comfort gets transmitted through that contact. And touch will mean more as each year goes by.

Stay Overnight in the Hospital with Your Confused Elder

If your mother has become disoriented or is in danger of slipping under stress into delirium, it would be best for someone close to her to stay through the night, talking softly to her, and reorienting her to who she is, where she is, why she's there, who you are. This might be the longest night you've experienced since your baby daughter was sick with pneumonia. Maybe the only thing the hospital has to offer you is a chair. Someone might be able to rustle up a cot if there's room. Around the world, mothers commonly sleep in the room of their hospitalized children and even prepare their meals and feed them to keep the thread of connection alive and well. Follow their lead.

Pay Attention to Basic Body Functions

The nursing staff looks after many patients and can't always be relied upon to monitor important areas of risk during illness (skin, bowel, bladder, balance). What can a family easily help with in order to ensure safe and appropriate care for a parent—the kind of care that won't put him or her back in an immediate crisis and perhaps force a return to the hospital shortly after returning home?

The most urgent issue, something that becomes a risk for complications within hours (yes, hours) of admission, is skin stress and breakdown. When an ill elderly person stops moving, in a bed or in a chair, fragile skin can very quickly start to show the discolored patches that can be the beginning of a pressure injury. Illness, poor overall health, poor nutrition, dehydration, damp or wet skin (often from unattended bladder incontinence): any of these makes things worse. Ask nurses to teach you about protecting skin health. You may have to be monitoring these conditions at home on your own very soon.

Transient urinary incontinence occurs very commonly during an illness or hospitalization. Sleep disruption, drugs, difficulty moving, and more fluids to process than the bladder had been accustomed to all contribute to this situation. Don't panic. This difficulty can be worked on and usually helped, but it may take some time. If a technical solution such as inserting a urinary catheter is suggested, be sure to ask a lot of questions about the pros and cons. Weaning an elder off a catheter may prove difficult. Slow Medicine urges the use, whenever possible, of tried-and-true, low-tech, labor-intensive aids: diapers, absorbent pads, frequent changes of clothing and bedsheets, frequent sits on the bedpan or bedside commode or trips to the bathroom. Moving around is always helpful. You were looking for something really useful to do. This is the kind of hands-on care that is the core of Slow Medicine's human rhythms and methods.

Pay attention to lazy bowels, or you will be faced with managing laxatives and enemas when your parent gets home. A little tea or coffee, prunes, or other favorite remedies brought in from the outside can help, but always check with the nursing staff first. The digestive system becomes lazy when it is given a chance to rest. Losing one's appetite is not uncommon during illnesses; all those medications going into an empty stomach certainly don't help. But it is important to get your parent's eating started up as soon as possible. He or she may resist and need some coaxing with favorite foods. Work with the nursing staff on this. Be aware that the insertion of a feeding tube is often an efficient shortcut that succeeds in getting the patient out of the hospital sooner, but simply shunts the problem of reestablishing eating onto your shoulders when your parent returns home. *Once an elderly person loses his or her appetite, it can take weeks or months to return.*

Finally, keep Mother moving. It is amazing how often the person making the decisions about discharge and disposition (home, nursing home, rehab) hasn't directly experienced what happens when the patient is actually asked to walk. You will be in a good position to bring your mother's mobility issues to the attention of the discharge decision-makers. Try to take several short walks daily with your mother on your arm (alone or with help from the nurse, so that you acquire the skill). *Let her hang on to you; don't hang on to her.* Her balance will be better (and better tested) that way. Over the next several weeks, as you ask her to take your arm for longer and longer strolls, chatting as you move along, you will be amazed at how sensitive an indicator of recovery her walking competency is.

BUILD YOUR ADVOCACY TEAM

Seek a Covenantal Commitment

If you have not already succeeded in doing so, have your most diplomatic family member speak with your parent's favorite physician now about the possibility of his or her becoming your parent's designated physician friend, committed to showing up and advocating for your parent during any and all such future crises. Slow Medicine relationships get established by requests far more often than by offers to help. It never hurts to ask for what your family needs.

Rally the Troops

Beat the bushes. Track everyone down. Twist some arms. If family members can't come immediately, put them on the telephone with Mother. Then negotiate when they will arrive. Chances are better for securing commitment during a crisis. This work also gives you a chance to spell out exactly what kind of support you yourself need. Is it sleep, child care, grocery-shopping, coverage while you keep other commitments? Or is it major emotional support?

Bring in the Reserves

Go out in search of the members of your parent's Circle of Concern, those friends and acquaintances who may not yet have heard what is going on. Elders have often developed extensive networks of connections over the years attending a church, book club, sewing circle, or activities at a senior citizen center. Or perhaps there's a friend who lives down the hall in your parent's apartment building, or a neighbor down the street. Simply let people know what has happened. Make some calls. Knock on a door. The news will spread. Past experiences with their own or other friends' crises make their pooled experience invaluable for support and problem-solving. There will commonly be many more people in this Circle of Concern than you expect. Remember, for elders without families, this "surrogate family" is the foundation of their support during a crisis.

Identify the Next Level of Your Team—Those Who Are Able to Stay On

It's Day Three, and the crisis is beginning to abate. Even if you don't feel this yet, the hospital team certainly does. If you have done your work and gathered together your parent's advocacy team, you now face the issue of who stays on. Everyone's reserves have run down. All those stress hormones and the adrenaline that surged through your body over the first few days to keep you going are now depleted. How do you start to address the question of who stays on? Get ready for the next round of negotiations.

Use Your Advocacy Team—You Can't Do It Alone

Call a family huddle—soon. Who can you ask, and how much can you ask of them? The doctors are talking about the medical care issues and sorting out how to carry out that part of the program. You are now faced with a weakened, frailer parent who is not ready to jump up and go it alone, although your parent may try to convince you that all he or she needs is to get back home and be left alone—a recipe for disaster. (Be aware that the medical care system counts patients' hospital readmissions as one of the indicators of inadequate quality of care, a good thing to keep in mind when you are negotiating to prevent too early a discharge.)

From the hospital's point of view, the acute crisis is passing, but immediate, and perhaps lasting, practical considerations are just beginning for the family and those in the Circle of Concern. How are you going to support your parent in the new condition and provide what he or she needs to get back to a steady state of compromise? Don't put on the blinders. Get down to work by reviewing your parent's activities of daily living (the AADLs or the IADLs) and then adding them to the care plan from the hospital. *If there is any chance to gain eligibility for some transition time in a supportive rehabilitation program, consider that.* Resist rapid overreacting and overcorrection. Curb the anxiety of family members who are prematurely pressing for your parent's permanent admission to a nursing home (what your parent is worried about right now) because they don't want to be bothered or can't stand the uncertainty of not knowing what to do. At this time of first crisis, think of any rehabilitation as an appropriate extension of a too-short hospitalization.

ENGAGE MEDICAL CARE

Narrow Your Agenda

You need to talk; they don't have time to listen. The medical staff and nursing staff are trying to focus on your parent's immediate care. You need to be involved. They sense that. But the situation often doesn't allow the time to accomplish everything you would like. How do you narrow your agenda so that it fits into their tight schedules? Look to the ancillary staff to help you learn and define what is happening and what is coming up. Ask to see someone from Social Services within the first day or two of your parent's admission. Ask for a preliminary visit with the discharge planner (who may or may not be part of Social Services). Talk as soon as you can with the physical therapist—who is usually activated very early to help with the movement toward early discharge. Remember the descriptive evaluation of your parent's capacities that you did back at the Station of Compromise? Retrieve those notes now. Let the therapist know what your parent's routine levels of function were before this illness. Go into the details. Seek consultation with the chaplaincy service. Don't worry about religious affiliation; chaplains are trained to listen and be helpful to everyone. All of these ancillary staff members will have a little more time to spend with you than the acute care team of nurses and doctors. Talking with them will give you a perspective that better prepares you for core medical discussions.

Resist Overly Aggressive Treatment and Its Hazards

Contemporary acute medical interventions are very good at stabilizing a difficult crisis. Often within hours there is perceptible improvement in an elder's condition. Dramatic improvement can result from a quick shot of intravenous (IV) fluids, for example, or the administration of a new drug. With younger, more resilient patients, it is often possible and desirable to go beyond mere stabilizing measures to take fairly aggressive action to correct a condition totally. *Beware of such promises for your parent. Elders in Late Life often do not have a physiology resilient enough to withstand aggressive interventions beyond what is needed to stabilize their immediate situation.* In this dangerous time of crisis, Slow Medicine's wait-and-see approach to treatment serves them much better.

Stay Focused on Getting Through the Crisis

Remember that the key to dealing successfully with a crisis is simply getting through it. This is not the time for an extensive examination of Mother's every little complaint (although that may seem tempting to you, since she has been so reluctant to seek help). This first crisis is best treated as a very focused intervention. Once you are through the crisis, a broader range of issues can be addressed. Many health care systems will prefer to follow up these other issues after the hospitalization. In academic settings where medical students and residents are trained, be prepared to address every possible issue (over and over). Exploration and repetition are great for training physicians, but may not serve your mother very well right now in that they muddy the waters, tire her out, and may lead to a lot of unnecessary testing. You may have to run interference or risk saying no to those earnest and eager students. What your mother needs now is focused care to get through the present illness. Incidentally, use your trusty notebook to keep a list of issues (her minor blood test abnormality, toenail and callus problems, persistent mild cough, unreliable bladder) that need to be followed when she returns as an outpatient. Others will have invariably forgotten these details.

Get to Know the Three D's: Depression, Dementia, Delirium

These three conditions often travel together, and all three slow and confuse thinking. If your parent suffered even mild confusion and disorientation during this crisis, go back to look for any telltale signs of decreased mental sharpness (memory problems, self-neglect, poor judgment, loss of interests) in the period before the hospitalization. A parent may have been especially at risk for an accelerating crisis without your knowing it. Your family and the doctors will benefit from your clear recognition of what was going on before the crisis struck.

How the Three D's connect is complicated. An elderly man who senses that he is losing the capacity to think quickly or well may begin to fear that he has dementia . . . and may then, quite understandably, become depressed. Depression, you will remember from your own intermittent experiences, can by itself slow thinking. Things turn over and over in the mind. Now your parent suffers a double whammy—mentally slowed and emotionally depressed. Adding the stress of a hospitalization to the fragile functioning brain of a person with *depression* and (even mild) *dementia* can produce *delirium*'s "veil of fog."

Take Advantage of New Teams

Often in the course of treatment, if one condition worsens more than others, a patient will end up with a whole new set of doctors in a different specialty. New doctors can bring a lot of energy and some new understanding to an elder's situation. Consider such a new development a high-risk, high-gain opportunity. If the new team shows itself to be focused predominantly on clarifying your parent's clinical situation, particularly by doing a lot of Slow Medicine thinking and deliberating, all well and good. But keep your ears open. If you hear suggestions for a whole barrage of "available" tests, be sure to ask for thoughtful and well-supported reasons. Because of your parent's present weakness, special tests that merely exclude conditions with a very low probability of being present may not be helpful here at this time. Be sure to get exact details on what each test involves (the physical requirements and negative side effects) and, thus, how such a procedure might further deplete your parent's stores. Could a test be as easily done two weeks from now, when your parent is stronger?

Medicine Concentrates on Diseases and Problems; Families Need to Focus on Capacities

The medical care team in the hospital is trained to uncover and define diseases, assess problems, and make recommendations for treatment; a Slow Medicine approach by the family (and sympathetic doctors) focuses on a parent's positive attributes and capacities: that is, setting forth what strengths Father has to call on as he begins the process of self-healing. *Medical therapies can correct and stabilize; they cannot heal.*

When the balance of the body is restored, it can begin its slow journey back to better health. Work with your father's team to mobilize his innate strengths for healing.

Be an Attentive Watchdog

Don't let anyone convince you that you are becoming paranoid when you monitor your parent's medications and other treatments and ask questions. It is not unreasonable to check the names of medications, doses, and reasons for their use. Getting an explanation that something is "routine" is not good enough. If anyone challenges your efforts, keep in mind this simple fact: in three days, after having been cared for around the clock by the nursing staff, your mother will be discharged and wheeled to the hospital entrance. Once she steps from the wheelchair into your car, clutching the return appointment slip to see her doctor in two weeks, *you are expected to take over all the functions that the highly trained and skilled nursing staff had, until just moments ago, been handling.*

It is good to start early in your preparations for this responsibility. With regard to monitoring medications, keep in mind the following: roughly half of all medication errors occurring in the hospital take place during the initial transcription into the hospital record of the medications and dosages that the patient had been taking at home. Many others occur when the writing of prescriptions and directions is done prior to discharge. *Careful vigilance and reconciliation of your parent's old medicine regimen with the new routines make for a high health payoff.*

When to Ask for a Conference

What about when things don't go so well in the hospital, or, even worse, start spiraling downhill? Sometimes the original reason for an elder's admission turns into a much gloomier picture. Stay calm. You are not likely to be the person to single-handedly reverse the course of cascading events (even though you have always been your parent's knight in shining armor). A sense of guilt and defensiveness at unexpectedly bad outcomes can set in very quickly, and communication between you and the staff shuts down. "We can't say anything just yet." Well, yes, and no. *Doctors and the staff can always help by sharing their thinking with you,* particularly if you can listen quietly and not critique their thinking before you have had a chance to live with their viewpoint for a while. After a day or so of this approach, it is okay to ask for a conference so that everyone involved can try to reconcile what may be conflicting views. This is part of all good medical practice and a key part of Slow Medicine practice—a real shared undertaking between the medical staff and families. In crises, there is a huge amount of uncertainty, and individual judgments vary. Keep on promoting everyone's engagement and reflection. Try to avoid having your own anxiety contribute to the problem. Review your parent's problems with the chaplaincy group. Its members have experience with hundreds of stressful situations and can offer support and advice. Once you are centered again, show up fresh at the bedside.

Addressing the Quick Discharge Problem

Watch out for the sudden discharge decision. Perhaps the hospital is short on beds or your parent has taken longer to stabilize than expected. "We think she could go home this afternoon." Whoa! Hold your ground. *Discharge planning should be a mutual task, and the receiving team needs to be prepared to accept the responsibilities that come with transfer of care to another location.* Do you know where your parent is going? Are all arrangements made and systems in order? Are you absolutely sure? Do the people on your advocacy team have their schedules coordinated? Who will accompany your parent to the next location? How will he or she get there? Be sure to continue to gather names, telephone numbers, e-mail addresses, pager numbers, and whatever else might be helpful in tracking down the hospital staff members who cared for your parent if problems develop after discharge. Do this even if your parent is going for a stay in a nursing home, because standard communications between hospitals and nursing homes are quite often woefully inadequate.

Avoid Premature Long-Term Decisions

This first crisis and hospitalization can provoke a premature decision for an elder's permanent transfer into a nursing home. All the elements are there—vulnerable elder, gathered family, available doctor—a dangerous combination for purely convenient decision-making. Beware the quick and easy decision to relocate your parent permanently. It can result in unhappy consequences for all.

HOW ARE YOU feeling? Coming out of the rapid trip through the world of acute medical care, you may be emotionally drained, or perhaps overwhelmed by what you are beginning to sense lies ahead. When that first telephone call came, telling you about the crisis, you may have felt some relief knowing that your parent was on the way to an excellent hospital—"Surely the doctors and nurses there will handle this well. It's what they do day in and day out." Perhaps you experienced a fleeting temptation to leave it all up to them. Surely they could handle the crisis so efficiently and effectively that you wouldn't even have to show up; you could simply provide support over the telephone. That would neatly get you off the hook and let you concentrate on your personal commitments and work schedule. Rationalizing is a common reaction, often coupled with pressured telephone calls to doctors and the hospital to make sure your parent is getting all the care the family feels is needed.

You may be telling yourself that this is just a onetime illness, and that your parent will get through it as easily as you survived your own pneumonia. Be aware of magical thinking. A more likely course is that this first crisis will turn out to be the vanguard of a recurring pattern of illness. Your elder's journey through the hospital provides a window into the many serious problems doctors and nurses face daily. So while you may be optimistic about your parent's immediate future as you leave the hospital, you will probably have to reconcile this optimism with your own unspoken intuitions and feelings about what lies ahead.

As an uncertified stranger in this new territory, you may also feel disempowered. This feeling may coexist with feelings of respect and deference complicated by strains of rebellion and detachment toward your parent, all of which may exaggerate your general discomfort as you take these first steps toward "sharing control."

At your mother's bedside, as you look at her lying there—spindly legs and bony shoulders, skin so thin—you realize that she has aged significantly. The hospital staff, sensing your distress and trying to comfort you, will remind you that your parent is getting older. In a very real sense, these doctors (mostly younger than you) are looking to you to decide how you want to care for your parent. You have now become an older adult caring for a very old parent. The life-cycle wheel has suddenly turned, and this can be quite depressing. And then your spouse asks, "What does this mean for my own parents?" And, "How are we going to balance their needs against your mother's?"

Tucked back in the recesses of your awareness may also be the early emerging understanding that this, too, will happen to you someday—sooner than you had ever contemplated before. So far, you may have seen your mortality reflected in rare episodes when contemporaries have accidents, early-occurring cancers, perhaps a heart attack; now you are forced to see, fleetingly, hints of your own future.

Recovery

"She'll be with us for a while."
—REHABILITATION NURSE

Bertha had been sleeping on our living room sofa since her arrival because she could not navigate the stairs, up or down, with the pain in her back and leg. At night, she rang a little bell, and my wife or I hurried downstairs to help her into a wheelchair, roll her to the bathroom, and help her onto the toilet. For modesty's sake, the bathroom door was closed while Bertha "did her business." Then we helped her to stand, eased her into the wheelchair again, rolled her back to the sofa, and tucked her in. If we were lucky, this would happen only once or twice a night. After two weeks, Bertha's healing was not progressing; she was barely holding her own. Everyone was getting tired. It was "time to have the talk."

Bertha sat in her wheelchair looking small and crumpled. This woman who had stoically endured so much during her life was very near to giving up. Did she have the hope, strength, and spunk to make another try at getting back to self-sufficiency? I sat on one side of her slumping form, and my wife sat on the other, "Bad Cop" and "Good Cop." I put the case: Despite the pain she was experiencing, if she didn't start a physical rehabilitation program very soon, Bertha might lose the opportunity for proper healing and be relegated to a wheelchair existence, forsaking her senior apartment and spending the rest of her days in a nursing home.

"Torturer!" the sweet woman moaned, unable to distinguish our concerned urging from sadism. Yes, the exercises would be hard work. Yes, she might at first find them painful. No, we were not trying to be mean. No, we didn't want to put her in a nursing home. She needed to understand that she was at a crossroads from which she might never return if she refused to invest the necessary energy and work with our help and encouragement right away.

After her crisis and spending two weeks in the hospital, much weakened by inactivity and using a walker, Bertha was discharged to her apartment, where it quickly became apparent that she was in no state to care for herself. She needed a wheelchair. Then our family, like so many other families I've attended, decided to launch upon a conservative middle pathway of care, our first steps along the trail to the final mountaintop. Rejecting on the one hand the easy despair that would sentence her to a wheelchair existence (some relatives called for her immediate admission to a nursing home) while refusing the other suggestions for dramatic invasive therapies (such as back surgery), I brought Bertha to our home to be cared for by us. We would see what rest, encouragement, and our personal hands-on involvement (supported by the efforts of a visiting nurse and physiotherapist) might do.

AFTER THE CONFUSING rush through the waters of a crisis, you will sense how relatively peaceful it is in the world of rehabilitation, whether it is undertaken at home or in a facility. Appropriately, more lengthy or intense programs require being in an institution. Populated for the most part by older patients with disabilities—some temporary, some with the makings of chronic burdens—this station is marked by slower movement. The hospital's stretchers, IVs, bedridden patients, and hurrying attendants are replaced by a much more leisurely appearing staff and a more mobile group of patients.

As a vigorous adult, you may take a while to get used to the variety of supportive devices being pushed and pulled around the halls and the more pervasive presence of human odors. Remember back to the arrival of a new infant when you first learned to accommodate your daily rhythms to the bathing, changing, and feeding routines, and the folding and unfolding of the latest newfangled travel gear. At this station of your parent's life, you will experience the need for the same kind of devotion. In our everyday lives, we aren't used to seeing so many people with striking limitations of function.

Still, this is a station where a feeling of optimism prevails. Rehabilitation professionals are the menders of the medical world, weaving small threads of strength together day by day, coaxing a little more out of beaten and wearied bodies. In a sense they are also the gardeners of health care, working to nurture and support natural healing. For most adult children, their first impression is that this is not a bad place to see your parent land. It is welcoming, and, after all he or she has been through, you'll probably feel relieved.

Going with your parent through the admission process at a rehabilitation center or filling out forms with a home care team, you will be pleased at the detailed assessments the physical therapists (lower-body workers), occupational therapists (upper-body workers), speech therapists, social workers, nurses, and physicians undertake. Upbeat, comprehensive, methodical, and less rushed than the staff at an acute care hospital, these professionals are great additions to your Slow Medicine team. You will most likely feel in good hands and become a little more relaxed and hopeful. Be aware that for both you and your parent, the timing of entry into this Station of Recovery coincides with a physical and emotional dip you may be feeling (now three to seven days from the start of the crisis). Your stress hormones have been depleted. You all have been running on the fumes in your energy tanks, and it is good to rest a bit. After a couple of days of being a little down, you will in all likelihood perk up, but the rebound will probably be slower for your parent. Everything is slower for him or her now.

After suffering all the stresses of crisis, besides feeling a physical letdown heralded by a loss of energy, strength, and appetite, an elder in Late Life will quite commonly experience a period of demoralization. "It feels all over. What a long way back! Sign me up for the nursing home." With our increased understanding that depression is a common problem with aging, there comes a temptation by many to give this momentary despair a label of "depression" and then jump immediately into drug treatment (with all its accompanying risks). Resist that response. Accept that elders' realistic understanding of the spot they find themselves in warrants some demoralized feelings, at least temporarily. Expect that during the first week or two after leaving the hospital these feelings are likely to be a part of your parent's experience. Support your parent through this transition by being patient and positive.

Rehabilitation is the near shore of the world of chronic care. Hidden inland from where you've touched down there is a whole world of institutional and community chronic care (assisted living, "rest homes," "bed and board," "grammie apartments"). You may discover this larger world later. But right now, a rehab program within the walls of a nursing home immediately suggests to your mother how close she is to a future life needing chronic care. When discussions started at the hospital about your mother's relocation upon discharge, you may have been told that she might or might not qualify for a full-fledged rehabilitation unit of the kind often located right at the hospital. For that, she would need to have the strength and stamina to participate in high-intensity therapy sessions, probably twice daily, scheduled in with younger patients—perhaps those recovering from strokes, perhaps those working on their rehabilitation after hip fracture repair or an elective joint replacement.

Given that your parent is older and subject to the increased frailties of Late Life, someone may suggest that he or she would be better off in a skilled nursing program (that is to say, in a nursing home) where a less demanding program of rehabilitation care might be more appropriate. Nursing homes often have a mix of "skilled care" patients (20 percent on average) and "nonskilled care," or "custodial care," patients (80 percent on average) in the same facility. Of course, if family members are involved and willing to provide hands-on support, there is the possibility of home rehabilitation—an option that spares an elder the vision of things to come. These alternatives represent very different levels of engagement and, thus, very different psychological perspectives for the elder and for the family.

All of this leads to perhaps the most important point I can make about the Station of Recovery: *it is an opportunity; don't let it slip away*. It is all too easy for an elder to drift from failed rehabilitation into needing further long-term chronic care. The clock starts right after the crisis, so don't take too much time out to rest. Rehabilitation is formal and demanding. If a patient is viewed as having the potential to regain capacities and functions lost through an illness or accident, rehabilitation care is paid for by Medicare—for a period of time (twenty days of full coverage, eighty days of partial coverage per episode)—either at a formal rehabilitation facility or at a skilled nursing unit or at home with rehabilitation organized through a home care agency. Nursing homes all try to attract rehabilitation patients because payment rates are higher for them than for patients needing "custodial care." Rehabilitation facilities and nursing homes also complete for the best patients (that is, cases that are straightforward and don't represent financial and clinical risks because of having a broad array of other problems that could go wrong or flare up).

Recovery in Late Life usually takes a lot longer than you may have been led to believe by hospital-based specialists. An older person has less physical (and perhaps less emotional) strength to begin with. Everyone experiences the need for extra rest following an acute illness; an elder may require extra rest for weeks or months. Persistence pays off, though. "The tortoise wins the race" holds truer for elders than it does for any other age group. Remember: elders can become fit by exercising for short intervals, as short as ten minutes at a stretch. It's the cumulative effort that counts. They may not tolerate a schedule that requires thirty to forty-five minutes of continuous effort and thus may feel as though they failed to meet the goals set for them. Inexperienced therapists may write off an elder with poor early performances in therapy as lacking the capacity to recover. Don't be daunted. For an elder over eighty, it's realistic to think in terms of six to twelve months (or perhaps never) to accomplish full recovery after a major crisis requiring hospitalization. However, even partial recovery matters in this all-important effort to return home.

If undertaken seriously and with much active emotional and logistical support, structured rehabilitation can open the door to the possibility of higher levels of both functioning and health than might have been present before your parent's crisis. Those of us in the medical profession know that many elders have allowed themselves to slip out of good health by neglect. Strength, stamina, mobility, and flexibility are lost because of insufficient daily physical activity. Isolation has led to emotional vulnerability and perhaps poor nutrition. Cognition is dulled by too much television and too few challenges for the mind and emotions, too little practical problem-solving, and too few personal interactions, even on the level of simple card or board games. Spiritual strength has been sapped by loneliness and separation from a world of larger possibilities. A motivated therapist working with a committed and energetic family can strengthen all of these foundations for health in ways that can be surprising.

For success at this station of vital opportunity, program professionals, family, friends, and other members of an elder's community and Circle of Concern must coordinate their unstinting support. A commitment of daily energies and positive encouragement by every caring member of your elder's advocacy team can instill the confidence that these goals are realistic. Show up and pitch in; the very hard work of rehabilitation, restoration, and recovery takes place over a very long time. Families cannot park a parent in a program and expect that the potential miracles will happen in their absence. And it may require "tough love" at times.

Jesse was in his mid-eighties when he had knee replacement surgery. Overweight, he enjoyed his beer and a sedentary life. He waltzed into the surgery expecting to get rid of chronic pain, but not fully appreciating that he was going to have to get fit and learn to walk again. After weeks in the rehab program, he was making little progress. The family was beginning to panic. Would Jesse end up in a nursing home? What would this mean for his wife, Julia, now home alone and in poor health herself? Eventually, overcoming her longstanding reluctance ever to criticize her husband of fifty-five years, Julia talked to the doctor. "He's always been a little lazy," she explained. "I think you're not pushing him hard enough." Faced with fear of the nursing home and the more aggressive prodding of the rehab team, Jesse finally committed to the challenge and worked his way home to a much more highly functioning life.

Practical Tasks at the Station of Recovery

PUT YOURSELF IN THEIR SHOES

Try to Understand the Combined Toll of Illness, Therapies, and a Prolonged Hospital Stay

It is hard for anybody at any age to go through a serious illness without a crisis of confidence. "Can I make it back home?" "I know I don't have strength in my legs to get down to the laundry." The loss of strength from four days of lying in the hospital bed, the fuzziness your mother feels from the medicines, and her breathlessness with the least exertion tell her that many things are holding her back. You can be glad at this point that you took such pains at earlier stations to familiarize yourself with the details of just how much housework she was doing and how far she could walk. If your mother was a little out-of-shape before, expect additional losses in all areas of fitness—stamina, strength, balance, and flexibility—and in mental sharpness following from demoralization and fatigue. On average, a healthy young person put on hospital bed rest loses 1 to 1.5 percent of measurable strength *daily*; an elder's losses run in multiples of those numbers. No wonder Mom is struggling to get out of the chair on her own—those arms and thighs just shrank by 20 percent. She's tired and needs more rest—true . . . as long as rest is balanced judiciously with a strengthening program to restore what she has lost. Is her chance of falling going up? You bet. She is three times more likely to fall after one month of bed rest.

Who Are Your Parent's Traveling Companions?

If your mother is a rehabilitation program inpatient, help her get situated beside some cheerful and positive-thinking partners. Don't let her get dragged down by watching and hanging out with those who are depressed or in very serious straits. Talk with the nursing staff about matching her with a compatible roommate. Scout for potential friends for her when you visit. The range of persons undergoing rehabilitation is vast. There are those patients with single diseases such as chronic heart conditions, emphysema, long-standing diabetes with complications, disabilities from cancer, and a group recovering from hip fracture. Another large group is composed of those whose rehabilitation work will be noticeably slowed by sensory, emotional, or cognitive problems such as visual impairment, depression, or dementia. Help Mom to understand that her circumstances are only temporary and that you are there to support her fastest recovery.

If your parent really gets down to work, he or she can be an inspiration to others. Get to know your parent's chosen buddies in rehabilitation. Besides helping your parent and you to deal with your anxiety about this stay, showing sympathy and interest in others deeply enriches the hours you spend at a facility by helping you to become a part of the support system—for patients and staff alike. What have their various experiences been? How do they measure their own progress? How do they cheer others on? Do they have goals that might be worked on in common with your parent?

Recognize the Difference Between Repair and Healing

Don't fall for the surgeon's rosy view that the faultless repair he or she just performed equates with recovery. The repair set the stage and got your mother going in the right direction. In order to achieve recovery, the actual healing following repair will require personal effort, skilled guidance, and, most of all, adequate time. The underpinnings of healing are partly physical (better nutrition, rest, exercising the whole body), heavily supplemented by emotional, social, and spiritual support. Your mom is way out of her usual comfort zone. She needs help to believe that improvement is possible even though she is older and the challenges are steeper.

Most patients end up being successful graduates of rehabilitation programs. Will everything get back to exactly what it was for your parent? Generally not. We're talking about greatly aged systems here, not the surging vitality of youth. But I have very often seen a wonderful kind of overshoot phenomenon whereby a successful rehabilitation program not only remedies a particular deficit but actually helps an elder develop new areas of strength for better living overall. A newly acquired stronger upper body may allow your mother to move around better. Generous emotional support may help her overcome the emotional drag that was holding her back and also realign her life of the spirit. Keep an open mind about what recovery means for each individual. The physical reason for coming to the rehabilitation program may be just the pretext for broader overall improvement.

Become Familiar with the Rules of Reimbursement in Rehab

Educate yourself about the ways the rehabilitation team thinks and plans and about the Medicare rules it has to play by, which are every bit as complicated as a chess game. Rehabilitation is an expensive, labor-intensive process, and your parent's Medicare coverage and supplemental Medigap insurance have strict guidelines about what they are going to pay for. The rehab team and the administrators behind it are looking carefully at how they can describe and code your parent's problems and progress for reimbursement. Detailed descriptive standards have been established for what constitutes adequate progress in rehab for a patient to remain eligible for support. By and large, late-life elders are disadvantaged by these rules (they heal more slowly and they were not part of the age group examined when the rules were set). Expect that your parent will not have recovered to his or her full potential before eligibility for formal financial support comes to an end. You can work with the team to better document your parent's improvement and then file an appeal with Medicare, but don't waste all your energy in that particular effort.

Keep in mind that most elders end up needing a *continuing informal program* in order to get to their maximum potential. Work with the rehab team to prepare for the period after they are no longer there to help. Collect copies of all their exercise instructions and insert them into your parent's personal health journal for the convenience of all. Buy the necessary elastic straps and ankle and wrist weights. You may want to use them yourself one day, or they can become part of a neighborhood lending library of elder health aids. When your parent loses eligibility for financial support but still needs an organized, disciplined, daily exercise regime, get the family and your parent's Circle of Concern to sign on. Plan from the very beginning to continue rehab at home.

Prepare Yourself for New Financial and Personal Costs

It is widely understood that a third or more of all health care expenses for elders are paid for out-of-pocket by elders and their families. As an elder moves farther and farther away from acute care toward the chronic care part of the health care spectrum, that out-of-pocket proportion increases. You will discover very soon, if you have not discovered already, that in our medical system there is simply less insurance coverage for chronic care. Direct financial costs may actually be the smaller part of the real overall costs, particularly to family and caregivers. Added logistical and emotional stresses affecting relationships, jobs, and other community commitments begin to mount when families undertake chronic care. There are transportation difficulties in getting frail elders to and from medical appointments; missed work; rescheduled meetings; interviews and arrangements for companions. This is a good time for a family to explore and discuss the details and costs of the medical model of institutional care as opposed to a social model for care at home. How do the costs and risks of Fast Medicine's antidepressant prescriptions compare with a trial of a few hours of paid companionship supplemented by some short-term visits from church members? Massage has been shown to decrease use of pain medication. How does the expensive purple pill for indigestion compare with better food choices and companionship at meals? How can these two differing resource models best be coordinated and balanced in your parent's particular situation? What are the trade-offs?

Revisit Advance Directives

After several years of trying diligently to get patients to carry out an annual review of their living wills and durable powers of attorney for health care, our geriatric team opted instead for an "opportune moment" approach—finding times when such a review was not merely an intellectual exercise and going through the motions, but rather a time when we really wanted to know where everyone stood when the chips were down. How are the designees who are formally delegated to step in and make decisions for your family actually doing under the stress of a crisis or an emerging chronic problem? Are they fully involved now? Will they be readily available, both physically and emotionally, for future crises? Call the family together and discuss whether or not you seem to have the right quarterback for the next (and potentially more serious) round with the medical care system.

STICK WITH THE PROGRAM

Allow for Personal Idiosyncrasies

When your parent moves from acute care (the hospital) to rehabilitative care, the family must work to supplement the formal record. As we saw during the crisis, the details of function, attitude, durability, and history that enrich our Slow Medicine understanding of an elder come through the gathered perspectives of family, friends, and the Circle of Concern. The rehabilitation team needs to understand these other personal dimensions in order to tailor their efforts and focus their work. Since these professionals work with, say, eighty-five-year-olds of widely varying capacities, they will be able to make their own physical assessments, but some capacities are not so easily delineated. It may be clear that Irene lacks balance walking around obstacles now, but they might not realize that she has been bumping into things for the past thirty years. Was your dad an athlete? Does he like a challenge? A goal to shoot for? Strengthen the case for your parent by filling in the personal details.

Consider Prior Hardship Experiences

What to expect from your parent on this go-around through rehabilitation will depend on how durable, tough, and stubborn he or she has been in getting through past difficulties. Your expectations of your parent's resilience may need to be modified as you come to understand that he or she really has led a very blessed life and hasn't actually faced the kind of hardships that require grit and perseverance. Some of the most difficult experiences with elder patients I have encountered are with those who have had mostly good fortune. Be patient with someone who hasn't before faced the need to work very hard physically and emotionally over an extended period of time. Introduce your parent around to elders who have been through a lot and let their stories serve as a guide. It is fruitless to berate someone into trying harder—just watch the rehab therapists gently cajole and persist when the going gets tough. We can all learn a lot from them.

Identify Other Health Problems

There is a natural tendency to get focused on the new problem or the new disease. (After all, wasn't it the reason this whole crisis came about?) Part of the work of rehabilitation is to devote adequate thinking to some of the other problems your parent might have as well. The reason? Small improvements in the way your parent's other problems are tended to might make the difference between overall success and failure at this station. Closer attention to diabetes management (through a specific diet, some weight loss, a better exercise routine, and close supervision of medications) might give your parent the shot of energy needed to have more stamina for the physical therapy he or she is doing to rehabilitate a hip. Finally getting your parent to invest in better glasses may improve downward vision and allow him or her to walk up and down stairs with more confidence. Get the rehab team to look at and pay some attention to the whole list of things neglected in the past. Marginal improvements here can pay off handsomely.

Negotiating the Plea to "Go Home"

"If you would simply let me go back home, I know I would do better." Your parent may also be magically thinking, "If I get home, that will mean everything must be okay." It's probably true that your parent would be happier and feel better emotionally in his or her own home. You must respect that. Meanwhile, the real problems and functional incapacities cannot be ignored. When you are confronted with this plea, focus on your parent's level of functioning. Set very specific goals that relate to what your parent will need to be able to do in order to return home successfully (that is, in a style that is consistent with what your parent's support system can actually deliver). Your parent will tell you, "I have always done that in the past" (make breakfast, bathe, get dressed). You will want to be sure that the rehab team has determined that he or she can in fact do these tasks in the present. In fairness, remember that you can never create a situation of "complete physical safety"—in your parent's own home or, indeed, in a nursing home (where falls also happen). Allow your parent some degree of risk. Discuss what your family can tolerate. Consult the wise elders in your parent's Circle of Concern to help achieve a balanced consensus. Recognize that self-direction and self-efficacy (people's sense that they can have some positive impact on their own life) are important foundations for overall mental and emotional health. Respect your parent's viewpoint . . . and negotiate a family compromise.

Realize That Attendants Are Not Servants

"It's been so long since I have had so much attention. I could get very used to this treatment." As improvement occurs and an interest in life reemerges, many elders come to enjoy being the center of all this new activity. Much better than being so lonely at home. Families, too, suddenly have others who care and provide comfort. Appropriate concern and caring are making everyone feel better. Wheel-in shower rooms; the comfort of good skin care done with gentle hands. Some conditions are much better than they were at home. "Couldn't Mother stay on? It's better for her. We could all use a little more of this." Although this sense of satisfaction is exactly what should be happening if staff members are doing their jobs well, keep in mind that *all care is, at its core, a gift given to promote healing*. Weaning your parent (and yourself) away from this position of benefit may not be easy. The staff will eventually promote more and more independence for the patient (and perhaps more dependence on the family), and you may find yourself resisting. Don't bite the hands that heal. Their work is to get you all through this transition. They teach; you carry on.

Getting Beyond Going Through the Motions

Watch Mother. Getting up out of an armchair requires almost every bit of her arm strength. She has to lift her whole body high enough to get her legs to do the final bit of work. How many pounds are those arms lifting? Notice how they tremble. Could she do that lift three times in a row? In order to recover from the very real strength losses she has suffered—slowly over time plus suddenly with the recent crisis—your mother is going to have to work at the top of capacity. You don't build new muscle working at 50 percent effort. Ask any strength trainer. Chances are your mother is not prepared for this high level of demand (nor may be some family members). In order to succeed in a rehabilitation program, she needs to do more than go through the motions. This will tire her, discomfort her, perhaps even make her whine a bit. Support those therapists as they carefully extend her limits. Get a sense of how you will need to carry on when she leaves the formal program.

Be a Patient Rehab Coach

How coachable was your dad at the peak of his interest in sports? Was Mother ever interested in athletics? How easy is it for you to improve your golf swing? Can you still ride a bicycle? Can you do it with comfort in traffic? Mastering specific exercises to strengthen special muscle groups requires abilities that may have been subtly lost in Late Life. Oftentimes, elders with early dementia lose both their sense of orientation in the larger world and their spatial orientation in their body. Being told or being shown (and then actually remembering) how to carry out a program of exercise can be exceedingly difficult. Body memories get established only through repetition and practice. It takes hundreds of repetitions to acquire new muscle memories. Get in there and do some patient coaching.

Focus on Mobility Above All

Some of what you will need to do is defined by the rehabilitation staff. Much of what you will want Mother to have when she ends up back home is a better set of routines. You can play an important part in helping her develop these new habits. *The absolute foundation for your parent's future resides in continuing mobility.* Lose that and he or she (and everyone) will pay the price. Whenever you are with your parent, take him or her for a little stroll. Want to talk? Walk while you talk. Help your parent to enjoy being on your arm strolling outside or down the hall or in the room. This doesn't have to be lengthy, but it has to be frequent. Put a sign on the door: HEALTH REQUIRES WALKING. Better yet, as your parent gets stronger, try a few stairs. Muscle strengthening depends on your parent's lifting his or her weight step by step, slow and easy. Say that your parent will "feel the quiver." *I am asking you to commit to assisting your parent to walk until he or she reaches the "can't-walk-any-longer" stage of life,* which will someday come. Don't let it happen prematurely.

Become an Expert on Function

Use this rehabilitation experience to start seeing the world through your parent's eyes. Every day consists of a series of little activities—bathing, dressing, moving around—that have suddenly become more difficult since the crisis. Get acquainted with the world of elder home renovations and "durable medical equipment," the technical term for many of these aids. In addition to the walking devices, there are grab bars, raised toilet seats, bath benches, intercom, and night lights to deal with. Kitchen stove use, electrical cords, and carpets that bunch and slip become safety concerns. Your job is all about crisis prevention—you don't want to go back to do a rerun with a hip fracture.

Working with Pain

Over the decade of the 1990s an important campaign was carried out to help health professionals recognize and deal more thoughtfully and aggressively with pain, particularly in elders. Out of this grew more effective treatment practices. This important focus on pain continues to be emphasized, particularly in institutions. As with all improvements, especially those taking on the rhetoric of a campaign, it is good to be aware that occasionally one can overshoot the mark and end up with some negative effects. Some of the work of rehabilitation will cause pain, especially in the hours or days after therapy is begun. This is normal and to some degree provides feedback that guides the program. Using enough pain medication or, better, Slow Medicine's alternative methods for dealing with pain (heat, cold, massage, relaxation, and reassurance are examples) is important. But stronger pain medications, while valuable, can sedate, diminish motivation, depress appetite, change rest patterns, and on and on. No one is asking your parent to be a martyr, but keep in mind that some pain can be an indication of progress—particularly those last few exercise repetitions that really tire the muscle and build the strength!

BUILD YOUR ADVOCACY TEAM

Working with the Rehab Team

Participating in a formal rehabilitation program may well be your first experience of working with a team in health care. More and more health care is being delivered this way. Hospitals have dozens of specialized teams, home health services work in teams, and every service, facility, or program in between will emphasize its team approach. Although some lip service is generally paid to "having the patient on the team" or "at the center of the team," it doesn't always happen. The added step of including the family (or other important supporters) on the team is even less often taken. This is where you come in. Knowing that this may be new institutional territory, you will need to be the one to take the initiative. Keep in mind that when the members of the rehab team disengage (as they always do), you and your team of family and friends will be left to carry on. You may not need to master the technical part of their work, but certainly you need to have a grasp of their perspectives and broad approach to problems particular to your parent's rehabilitation. While it may be difficult to schedule an official meeting time with the entire team, it is appropriate to ask for regular updates from one or another team member. Almost invariably, asking for summary reports or requesting permission simply to sit in on a portion of a meeting will improve the overall quality of what you can communicate to family and friends.

Brief the New Arrivals—Theirs and Yours

As we have seen, the formal medical record will probably not capture what is most important about an elder's character and personality, history, habits, strengths, and weaknesses. Whether a new therapist is providing weekend coverage in the program or a new friend is recruited from a Circle of Concern, remember to do a short briefing. You need to be the go-between for any new people appearing on the scene to help out. Health professionals and informal supporters alike will benefit from and feel helped by your briefing. Quite understandably, many caring and willing but uninformed friends stay on the sidelines because they don't know exactly when or how they might be of help. Give them some suggestions about how they might contribute and solicit their advice. Reach out. Share your garden vegetables. Bake some cookies. Little things can affirm a sense of connection.

Identify Cheerleaders

By this time, your advocacy team contains a range of talented persons. Look for the cheerleaders. During a crisis, when an elder may be feeling overwhelmed and without hope, the "sis-boom-bah" approach may not be appealing. However, during rehabilitation, when hope is revived—though the game looks long and your parent is tired in the first quarter—bring your best and brightest cheerleaders onto the field. Unflagging, optimistic support is required once the rehabilitation process is engaged. Forget about being reserved. Get folks to cheer, especially when the therapist is driving Mother toward "peak performance." Keep an eye out for stories of success among the other patients—they can be very credible cheerleaders, having "walked the walk."

Stay on the Right Side of "Helpful"

As a family member or as a part of a Circle of Concern, the more sophisticated you become in your advocacy, the more you can contribute. Taking on this role for an elder is of immeasurable value. But remember, you don't want to come across as a threat to any of the health professionals you are working with. Rehabilitation teams can form close relationships with families over time. However, if you end up being seen as too demanding or pushy, even if these responses stem from your enthusiasm and concern, your team will disengage. Be careful not to let this happen.

Think of Your Own Health

It has become widely known that substantial risks to personal health, including risk of serious illness, are associated with the stresses of being a caregiver. The practice of "caring for the caregiver" is gaining increasing prominence. The period of rehabilitation offers an excellent opportunity to understand and acknowledge the sacrifices made and burdens borne by those providing long-term support. As family, friends, and others from a Circle of Concern begin to share their stresses and stories of caregiving, there is a chance now to begin to work on future practices of self-care, including time off and attention to one's own health foundation habits and medical problems.

Speak the Unspeakable

The balance for your parent may be shifting so that a major change of support and care providers may be on the horizon. It is never wrong to consider a nursing home option (a conversation conducted preferably without your parent's being present—especially initially, while the hopes of rehabilitation are being fueled). "Breaking the ice" on this taboo subject may prove helpful later. An assisted living community or nursing home may well become a part of meeting future care needs. These initial discussions open up new emotional territory for a family and will benefit from being processed slowly. Although broaching this issue will almost always make someone in the family want to bolt toward the "nursing home option," most families try to put this choice off as long as possible. At this time, simply get used to "speaking the unspeakable" as a way of sounding the depths of everyone's anxieties and commitment.

ENGAGE MEDICAL CARE

Try Not to Let Benefits Drive Clinical Care Plans

Much of how both providers and consumers think about medical care has been conditioned over many years by "what gets paid for by insurance." However, from an elder care perspective, things have gone astray, and many geriatricians have come to understand that designated benefits don't match their patients' needs very well. The fact that a particular service is not paid for by the Medicare program doesn't mean that it isn't helpful, or sometimes even necessary, for your loved one. During the rehabilitation period, you will hear things said about your parent's benefits—qualifying for them, limiting them, extending them. Don't confuse this talk with what Mother's real needs may be. You can see that though she is walking longer distances, she still doesn't have the strength to go up the six steps that take her to the bedroom. Your parent hasn't yet tested his or her balance and dexterity with food preparation. Coordinate your knowledge of your parent with the rehab team and personalize goals. Argue for their practical importance when your parent gets back to his or her own home and particular circumstances. You can be of considerable help to the rehab team in developing a fair plan—fair to both your parent and the insurance carriers.

Ask for Periodic Medication Reviews

Why is this medication being used? Is there still a need for it, given the progress that Mother has made? What does she think about its effects and value? Its side effects? Does she like it? Is it considered a necessary part of a long-term plan? Is there actual evidence that this particular medication is likely to have real value for her? How much, really? How is the medication being monitored? How should it be monitored? Could she try a lower dose or perhaps go without it for a trial? What are the risks with it? Without it? Could the way it is being given each day be simplified for her sake? Are there alternative therapies with fewer risks

and lower costs that might substitute for this medication? The rehabilitation program or nursing home is paying for your parent's medications now. Do you know the costs of each medication? Can your parent
(or you) afford these costs when he or she leaves the program and you
assume responsibility? Geriatricians are very aware that elders are in
general overprescribed to. The more medications, the more risks the
patient faces. In fact, *many hospital readmissions for elders are related to
medication problems.* One can never pay too much attention to reviewing
medication use and eliminating unnecessary or low-value-for-the-cost
prescriptions.

Prepare for the Next Handoff

In rehabilitation, the pace may seem slow at the beginning, but time
will fly by, and the end may come very abruptly. Have you thought about
how to connect to the next appropriate group of health professionals
who will assume your parent's care? There is going to be a complex
story to tell. The rehabilitation team will put together a brief summary
of what they have accomplished medically, but it will not come close to
describing the "inner journey" your parent has taken. Your Slow Medicine understanding of your parent's fears, hard work, setbacks, gains,
and all accomplishments that are leading him or her back to an independent life will seldom be found in those formal clinical notes.

Nor will this summary forecast in adequate detail what it really will
be like for your parent to function in a home setting. Remember that
you are the carrier of the real record—details of what capacities were
lost in the crisis and what strengths and weaknesses have emerged. If
you have paid close attention, you will know a great deal more now
about your parent's coping mechanisms, psychological state, and philosophical outlook.

As your parent's formal support team disbands and he or she heads
back toward the world of one-on-one medical care with a doctor, is
there any way of enlisting a new team to take the handoff? Establish

contact with the staff at your parent's doctor's office and undertake a more detailed exploration than you may have made in the past. Is there a nurse-practitioner or physician's assistant in the office? How many nurses? What do they do? Do they help coordinate care and communications? Is the office affiliated with a visiting nurse or care manager program? It is unlikely that this next team will come prepackaged. You will have to be the glue to make it a functional unit and to engage and alert the office-based medical team anew to your parent's changed situation. Do this successfully and you will be on the road of Slow Medicine, creating a new support system and security (physical, emotional, and psychological) in your parent's new circumstances.

Half a lifetime ago, in traditional community practice, a family's doctor would have eased this transition with some house calls to make sure all was going well. Although still in their infancy, new programs for home visiting by doctors and nurse-practitioners are being started in some communities. Check out the possibilities where you live (www. homecaredoctors, etc.) These programs will grow as their value is recognized by elders and families. If no such program is available in your parent's community, try to negotiate a house call from his or her regular doctor. It never hurts to ask, and it makes the medical community more aware of this important Slow Medicine need.

Look into Emergency Call Systems for the Home

Over the past decade a new technology, Lifeline, has been developed to help elders living alone. The best of these programs now have alarms worn on the body (bracelets or necklaces) that are easy for the wearer to activate. Memories of her time stranded in the bathtub made it attractive to my mother, Bertha. Your parent may need some coaching to convince him or her to use it. The key is to choose a Lifeline service that responds to an alarm that is acceptable to your parent and to your family. The first call doesn't have to go to the police station, the ambulance, the hospital, or the doctor. The best systems have telephone attendants who can listen via an in-home monitor and have a conversation with an elder in need to assess a situation further before initiating a call to the designated family member or neighbor—someone who knows your parent's situation intimately and who will immediately go to see him or her. Used early and well, these devices reduce the risk of precipitating an unnecessary crisis and transport to the hospital. Don't put in place a plan that removes control from your parent, or he or she may be reluctant to use it.

Prepare an Emergency Information Pack

A conversation with the local emergency responders who will serve your parent in time of need may be helpful. Ask what their experience has been with elders who live alone. Get their advice on preparing such things as an emergency information pack, which will hold (hopefully current) lists of health problems, medications and dosages, your parent's doctor's name and telephone number, and family members' names with telephone numbers and addresses for contact. Also get advice on where to store the pack so that the rescue team will know where to find it. Make regular updated copies for all family members and friends who may be a part of your responding group. When your parent returns home, pay attention to putting these important systems in place. *The one important event you must prepare for now is the next crisis.*

Taking Stock

At this time, you may be feeling a steady emotional urge to disengage . . . or at least keep your distance. "Now that the acute part of her illness is behind her, perhaps we can leave her ongoing recovery to others. She has promised to do her exercises daily." We want to support a return to more independence for Mother as soon as we can, and we quietly hope for our own escape back to life as we had known it. You may find yourself going back and forth in your search to understand your own motives. Still, uncertainty and accompanying anxiety have entered your life in a larger way. The rehabilitation program measured your parent's progress more formally in terms of distance walked, weight lifted, meals consumed—specific information to ground and comfort you. You will now need your family's informal yardsticks for measurement within your parent's own home and your own complicated life to gauge how your parent and you are doing from day to day. Imagined scenarios begin to play. "What will we do if Mother can't handle the stairs? What about getting out to shop?" Your parent's course in recovery will now be determined by his or her intrinsic strengths, hard work, luck, and the quality of caring by family and, more distantly, health professionals in their places of work. At some time during rehabilitation, all the uncertainty and anxiety provoked by the crisis abruptly shifts from your parent to the family. Your own emotional course will depend on how you and others negotiate each family member's involvement. What is your parent's changing role in making decisions—"Where am I going next?" "Who makes the decisions here?" You may see your sibs in sharper focus—the rescuer, the weeper, the prince or princess, "still the baby," the martyr. Where do you fit in? How will you deal with each other the next time around? "If you want to keep Mother at home, you take care of it." "Since you live the closest, perhaps you could start out the home support program." "If I provide more financial support, could you make the time to be with her?"

By now you have probably accepted the reality that there is a lengthy road ahead. As you embark on the rest of your shared journey, a lot will depend on how maturely you nurture your family relationships, your own emotional life, and your spirit.

Decline

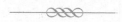

"We can't expect much more."
—VISITING NURSE

BACK AT HOME

After a crisis requiring three solid months of daily rehabilitation in
our home, it was amazing to think that Bertha could live alone in
her apartment again. We were feeling proud of the hard work we
had done and pleased to have been confirmed in our approach to
her care. In truth, however, the strength in her legs never really returned. There would be no more solo walks to the library. No more
going up or down a stairway by herself. Votes were split in the
extended family about the wisdom of her returning to live alone in
her senior apartment. Part of our plan at this early stage of the
Station of Decline was surely based on wishing—wishing for
Bertha's sake that she might once again live the life she wanted.
Happily, amazingly, that's exactly what she did for nearly two
and a half years—until the next crisis came on.

In the course of supporting her during that intervening time,
we begged her doctor not to do anything new or different without

making us aware of potential pros and cons. Yes, she now needed some help with bathing, one of those important ADLs, but Bertha continued to think of such help as optional. She promised to continue her exercises. She rather liked the fancy new red walker we got her to use outside the apartment. The cane (she promised us) would steady her when she moved around inside. She was happy. However, it became more difficult for her to tell a bill from an advertisement, and the workings of her telephone seemed more perplexing.

As food piled up in her refrigerator, we wondered about her nutrition. Helpful neighbors noted her need for more laundering of bedclothes, given her worsening incontinence. There was that disturbing refusal of the bus driver to let her ride to the mall . . . something about a fall while trying to get on. Bertha was mum about that. She took more naps and slept later in the mornings. We kept up our attentions by regular telephone calls and intermittent visits, but so much else was going on in our own lives. My sister's grandson was chronically ill and needing her time and energies; I became acutely ill and had to take leave from work. All the threads holding Bertha up were pretty slender.

In time, an unreported—and consequently untreated—urinary tract infection quickly sent Bertha downhill into a state of delirium. Three untended days of severe incontinence nearly destroyed her apartment, and Bertha had to be hospitalized again. The fragile balance of her health had tipped a second time. Bertha's strange failure to call for help before things got so out of hand shook everyone's confidence in her continuing good judgment. Clearly, her physical and mental capacities had declined more than we supposed. Now she needed more help to care for herself, and would never return to the Station of Compromise.

. . .

A SHIFT BEGINS, even if you have done your work well. This change arrives despite the admirable care and persistence with which you have worked to maximize capacities, improve strength and functioning, manage separate diseases, balance treatments, and avert possible crises. An aging body slips away a little more every few months or years. Finally, Mother has suffered losses significant enough to constitute real "disability," meaning that she can no longer live a "normal" life. The goal of aging well is to extend quality living as far as possible before disability eventually and inevitably arrives. This is the paradox of escaping earlier threats to one's health. If people live long enough, they will get to a point where, for example, they can no longer dress, bathe, use the toilet, or feed themselves without help. Incremental, unavoidable changes during the Station of Decline carry an elder over the threshold from "disability-free" to "disability-burdened." At age eighty, an elder with an average life expectancy of ten years will, on average, experience seven and a half disability-free years followed by two and a half years of being disability-burdened.

ANOTHER RESURRECTION

Bertha was angry that we refused to let her go back to her own apartment straight from her month recovering in assisted living from urinary sepsis. She was happy to be brought from Upper Michigan to our home for a month of observation and evaluation, but when the talk began about the family's plan to have her return to assisted living, she was fiercely opposed. This ordinarily mild-mannered woman tapped her index finger hard on the table to emphasize her opinion that she could look after herself. When we countered with her failure to let someone know she was sick before things fell apart so badly, she just shook her head and clammed up stubbornly. Did she want to come and live with us? No, that's not what she wanted. Okay, my sympathetic wife offered, maybe, like the last time, there was still a middle way. Perhaps, with enough additional hands to help, she could remain in her own apartment a while longer—for the summer, say—and then return to assisted living for the winter, the way her roommate there routinely did.

So began Bertha's "second resurrection"—a three-month trial that extended for fifteen months. My sister negotiated with two younger seniors in Bertha's apartment building who had unofficially been doing her laundry. For a modest wage, they signed on for daily duties and further oversight. Dear, dear Fran and Hazel! Two members of Bertha's local Circle of Concern stepped in to help her stay in her home a little longer. Utterly reliable, alternating days and weekends, they laid out Bertha's clothes each morning (she was still able to dress herself); made breakfasts, lunches, and dinners in her apartment; occasionally escorted her to Bingo (she could no longer keep up with the pinochle players) or drove her with her walker to church; gathered her mail; oversaw the proper loading of her pill-boxes and saw that she took the right medications at the right times; did light shopping and tidying up; helped her with bathing and her diaper for the night. They also telephoned my sister or me when they had concerns or noticed some change in Bertha's health or cognition. They were angels, to be sure.

The View from Here

The Station of Decline is a slow drift down a widening river. Eventually that river will empty its elder traveler into a limitless sea, but that may still be a very long way off. Month by month, year by year, during this drift of slow separation, the generations' worldviews shift and diverge.

Differences of perspective between elder, family, community, and medical care system grow. My view no longer coincides so well with my mother's. Her doctor is on distant "standby." How differently we experience this station.

In the Station of Decline, an elder's gradual separation becomes increasingly apparent to all. The river widens, and the busy world on the banks recedes. Along with Mother's failing hearing and eyesight come less penetrating interest and understanding. Recent events, politics, what is happening in the community, down the street, or next door are simply of less interest. The close-at-hand becomes most engaging: immediate details of living, the near view out the window, the motions of getting through each day. Perhaps some card or letter arriving in the mail, a magazine, a favorite TV program, devotional readings, a bouquet of flowers, or little present brought by a recent visitor attracts an elder's attention. "What the weather's like today," "what I had for lunch," and "how I slept" are central topics for conversation. Life is greatly simplified. Daily demands on cognitive skills decrease. Abbreviated communication arcs back and forth from shore to boat. Often family members feel as though they are calling but getting little or no response. What your mother reports on doesn't change much day by day, and what you report on from your world seems to interest her less and less. She doesn't really seem to want the details, just some reassurance that everyone is okay. Still, checking in remains a vital thread.

At this point the river seems broad and unmoving as a lake. Family and friends standing on the bank day after day may be unable to sense any perceptible change in the elder's course. There is more uncertainty about what might best be done to help. Though we are working hard to maintain her where she is, literally and figuratively, Mother isn't able to sustain her rehabilitation gains. Mere acts of will and effort are not enough. We may even discover that asking too much of her actually seems to undermine her health. Even our ritual of taking brief walks together has become too much.

THINGS FALL APART AGAIN

Bertha's legs stopped moving. For irregular periods of time they suddenly stopped responding to her thoughts, and her caregivers caught her frozen mid-room, teetering toward a fall. She began suffering little strokes. Withdrawn and without speech for hours at a time before "waking up," she was unaware of her absences and the fear and worry they caused her caregivers. Knowing that Bertha did not want "heroic measures," and valiantly refusing to subject her to an upsetting and exhausting emergency room experience, Fran and Hazel called to let us know her status, and then sat with her, observing her carefully, monitoring her breathing, waiting to see if she would wake again from any number of lapses.

Finally, after many months and years of working to keep Bertha in her own home, we exhausted all our resources. Our family's shared Late-Life journey required Bertha's transfer to a nursing home. On our way there, my ninety-one-year-old mother confessed that she had hoped and prayed each night to pass in her sleep before this hour came. I told her we all had prayed for a quick and peaceful deliverance for her as well, but none of our prayers succeeded.

After having been so loyally dedicated to helping your parent stay at home, even with all the benefits that have come to him or her through your hard work, your commitment, and your sacrifice, a time will often arise where there is nothing more you can do other than change course. You have exhausted your resources. Softened somewhat by your satisfaction at having worked so hard for so long, a painful pressure nevertheless builds when all your family's efforts finally reach their limits. Your loved one may simply need more care. A relocation to assisted living, a residential care facility, or a nursing home becomes the only answer for many, perhaps for most who are lucky enough to have parents who have lived long lives.

Having walked this pathway with families many, many times, I continue to be surprised by better-than-expected outcomes when a family's preceding efforts have been exhaustive and heartfelt. Mother is naturally unhappy at first to leave all she holds familiar. Who would not have such feelings? A transition that is forced or premature can prove difficult, even destructive. Guilt, disappointment, blame, and anger may all complicate such a transition. If the transition is well-timed, however, a deeper acknowledgment of necessity eases negative feelings for everyone. Furnishing your mother's new setting with familiar possessions can be an excellent "thread to the past," and the change may actually bring with it new energy in Late Life.

Mentally, Dan was still sound, but physical frailty forced the difficult decision to unburden his wife by moving him to a nursing home. Fortunately, the facility was only a couple of miles from their home so she could visit every day—and their sons with regularity.

One day two months on, when the sons arrived for a visit, he "shushed" them. The radio was on, and he was intent in his listening. When the music ended, he apologized and said, "For the first time in my life I have the opportunity to learn about music—that piece was so important to Beethoven's development."

———

It was a sad day when Lily's mother, Mary, had to leave her home of fifty-eight years. Mary wanted to live with her daughter, but no one could be home during the day to care for the eighty-eight-year-old elder's needs. Mary just knew that she'd hate the assisted living quarters after having kept her own home for so long.

What a surprise one month after the transfer when Lily called, to find that her mother was "out and about" in her favorite new spot, the bench outside the dining room where she could chat with every new friend who came by.

The Station of Decline is not only about the decline of an elder. It is also the story of a decline in the family—a decline of energy, resources, freedom, and latitude in one's own life. There is a sacrifice, a price to pay for this intimate, difficult, and rewarding experience of traveling the late-life path with your aging parent. Some cultures value and take enormous pride in fulfilling these filial devotions. Others experience great difficulty balancing this effort with personal needs, family, work, and financial obligations. In our culture, a reassessment of the value of this family caregiving is under way as more and more of us are forced to respond to the growing numbers of elders and the scarce public resources allocated for their care. Baby Boomers have begun to wonder how we ourselves may be cared for when we grow old. What we do now to and for our parents establishes patterns of concern and commitment (or neglect) that will carry forward into our own futures and the lives of our children.

As patterns of diminishment become established in the life of your elder, you may also begin to notice that the medical care system has been disengaging. The flip side of "We can't expect much more" is often "There's little more we can do." What this euphemism means is that under our current Medicare insurance schemes doctors are not paid adequately to do the kind of Slow Medicine attending that so many elders need at this time of their lives. We quite simply don't have enough trained internists, family physicians, and geriatricians to provide this vital care. This disengagement by Fast Medicine will be more complete in some instances than others. Part of the role of family, friends, and the Circle of Concern now will be to preserve links with health care professionals. It is much more difficult for elders with a "closing in" worldview to sustain these outside relationships and dialogues on their own.

Routes of Decline

THE LUCKY ONES

We all hear stories of "lucky" elders dying unexpectedly but peacefully in their sleep. Many wish for such an uncomplicated passing, but fewer than one in ten elders are spared a longer decline.

DEATH BY EXHAUSTION

Heart, kidney, lung, and liver failure are common pathways of decline in Late Life (about a third of all deaths, with heart failure the most common). At one time, vital organ failure led to a fairly rapid decline and death. A couple of decades ago, for instance, the prognosis for a major episode of congestive heart failure was as dire as that for aggressive cancer—a high likelihood of death within one year. Now, however, with better end-stage treatments available for cardiac, lung, and liver conditions and widespread availability of kidney dialysis, the usual trajectory for this route of decline is a slow downhill course with multiple acute crises.

For elders in Late Life, however, as diseases progress and treatments become less helpful, organ failure often leads to what I would term "death by exhaustion." There is simply no energy left for an elder to carry on. From the patient's and family's perspective, these late-life downhill courses are often characterized by very fragmented care involving many specialists and hospital treatments as well as the family's painful and growing uncertainty about medical decision-making. With problems of organ failure, there seems no end to what procedures might be, and are, offered for trial by doctors and hospitals. In the Station of Decline, the important question becomes: How much "life energy" does my parent have, first to endure the treatment and then to direct it

toward getting well? As the real value of new treatments becomes uncertain, deciding when to stop is very difficult.

> Misfortunes came early in Elizabeth's life. Her rheumatoid arthritis
> had already reduced her to a walker and wheelchair existence be-
> fore heart disease came along. She became one of the "prematurely
> aged" as her diseases advanced. Nothing worked. By her third hos-
> pitalization in the cardiac care unit, the prognosis was, "She's going
> to die very soon, perhaps within days. Would she like to be at
> home?"
>
> We settled her in the nursing home after a short failed trial at
> home alone with her husband, frail and not a man of action him-
> self. Elizabeth chose to have all her medications stopped except
> those that she felt clearly made her more comfortable, only one
> of which turned out to be a cardiac medication. Actually, this new
> life became sweeter for her. Her appetite returned. Many friends
> and family members visited. Four months passed. Finally she be-
> came more tired. It took another month before she felt she did
> not have the energy to eat or get through another day. A couple
> of weeks more and it was over.

Strokes

Injuries, both large and small, to the aged and fragile brain from ob-
structed blood vessels and the resulting complications of these inter-
ruptions of circulation remain very common causes of disability and
death in late life. Strokes disable elders more often than they kill. Large
strokes bring immediate, often major, disability. Yet small strokes of
the sort my own mother sustained (many brief or barely perceptible in
their effects until they began to accumulate in number) also lead to a
loss of capacities and progressive disability. The downhill path of decline from strokes is slower than that of organ failure and usually involves fewer major acute crises. As well, strokes often mix in with the

brain changes of Alzheimer's disease, and together the two conditions create a very gradual and prolonged downhill path.

Cancer

There are, of course, many different kinds of cancer, some curable, some very treatable, and some still deadly. Many cancer experts would point out that elders are likely to have many undetected cancers that they "die with, not die from." Prostate cancer in men is the most widely cited of these. Others would be hard to detect, except at autopsy. Today, successful cancer treatment can turn what once was a relatively quick passing into more chronic illness and decline to death over a period of time that may last months to years. In midlife, the common "pattern" of cancer deaths (assuming that treatment secures a temporary remission) shows a very high continuing level of function and health after treatment, followed by a fairly short, precipitous decline to death when the cancer becomes uncontrollable.

When cancer comes to a person in late life, however, the extended prognostic trajectory of "high functioning and good health" may not hold so true. Because of general physical vulnerability, lower resilience, complications from other significant medical problems, and the deleterious impact of demanding treatments, many elders experience a much reduced level of health during and after cancer treatments. Many cancer treatment specialists have begun to recognize this fact, and a subspecialty of oncology is emerging that specifically focuses on the special problems of cancer treatment in elders.

Priscilla's neighbor, a public health nurse, telephoned to ask if I would stop by. Everyone seemed a little embarrassed because a doctor's visit was long overdue. The patient and her husband had been hoping for an easier course. In their late eighties, they knew that the wife's cancer meant the end. I had seen the living arrangements before: all the rooms closed off except the kitchen and the adjoining living room, the bed moved downstairs to save on heat. The air was close and smelled of illness. They didn't have much money and feared the hospital, said the friend and neighbor who had agreed to help care for Priscilla at home, since they had no children. When I unwrapped the turban of cloth around her breast, the fulminating tumor bled readily. She was quite weak from slow blood loss over months. But she hadn't died, and now it was too difficult to keep up with the nursing. They were all feeling that their well-intended plan was becoming a neglect they couldn't tolerate. What could I suggest? Here started the cascade of best intentions: we would find a surgeon, do minimal surgery to make the wound care easier, return her home to die. When the unexpected small stroke she suffered in the hospital added too much to the burden of her care, she had to be moved into a nursing home. There went their savings and the house. Her husband moved into town for the short time he lived after her death.

Physical Frailty

There have been, and continue to be, some physicians who declare that "people die of diseases, not from aging." I wish one of them were with me when I repeatedly struggled to identify a distinct "cause of death" for a death certificate of an elder with advanced frailty. Recently, geriatricians have worked to define "frailty" more specifically. One study looked back through medical records for causes of death in a large group of elders over eighty and estimated that nearly a quarter of the time, it would have been more accurate to ascribe the cause of death to frailty than to any specific disease.

Frailty could be called the "unmeasurable disability" because it can often develop and advance without the loss of specific ADLs or IADLs associated with more defined disabilities. Slowly, the older person loses physical strength, stamina, speed of movement, sensory capacities, and overall energy. Most elders in this position can still bathe, get dressed, move about, use the toilet, and eat independently, but these activities absorb so much of the day's energy that relatively little is left for anything else. Such decline follows a very gradual (usually over years) downward path. With good care and barring bad luck, the aged body slowly shrinks like a leaf in autumn. Eventually, a minor illness or "giving up" tips the balance, and death ensues.

Dementia

Alzheimer's disease, vascular (or small strokes) dementia, Parkinson's-associated dementia, and other degenerative brain disorders can run courses ranging from extremely slow (one to two decades) to rapid (two years to death). A general trajectory of decline from dementia has been difficult to describe. There are many physically vigorous elders with advanced Alzheimer's disease who lose their health only when other diseases come along. However, we know that eventually Alzheimer's and these other dementias become terminal conditions, causing so much brain damage that death ensues because of progressive loss of physical functioning (movement, speech, ability to eat). Occasionally, barring intervening infections (to which elders become very susceptible), brain disease leads to seizures and death. After age eighty-five, dementia becomes progressively common, and its predictable course usually involves more than one of the other described patterns of decline.

My friend Alice called with a "technical question" about advance directives. Her father had been in a special dementia unit of a nursing home for nearly three years and was now in advanced decline. Her mother had called to say that the nursing home was sending him to the hospital, ill with pneumonia. Alice and her brother lived hundreds of miles away from their parents. "We did the advance directives last year, and a copy was filed at the hospital. Do they need an original?"

Like so many of us, Alice thought that filing advance directives for her father meant that they would automatically be found and followed. "It might be best to head there yourself," I advised. Alice and her husband were there by the next morning, having alerted the hospital staff in the meantime by telephone about her father's expressed wishes for no "heroic measures." He died peacefully within two days. The hospital recorded "pneumonia" on his death certificate, though the family felt he had died of dementia years before.

Decline, But Where?

An elder's slow journey of decline may unfold in many different locations: an original family home, a downsized senior apartment, the back bedroom of a family member's home, an assisted living facility, or perhaps a nursing home if other housing situations have failed. Your mother naturally prefers to stay in her familiar boat, and you would like as much as possible to keep her there. That sense of home means a lot, providing emotionally and psychologically secure space, particularly if you are detecting some small failures of cognition and slips in behavior.

We live at a time when housing options in Late Life are expanding rapidly. This is driven in part by the commercial opportunities created by burgeoning numbers of elders over eighty years old—the group most likely to need supported living arrangements as they age. At any given time, only about 20 percent of those over eighty-five years old reside permanently in nursing homes. Eighty percent remain in their own homes or the homes of family members or in group living arrangements. For those aged seventy-five to eighty-five years, only 5 percent live permanently in nursing homes. The real crunch on nursing home bed capacity has come about because of the present growing numbers of elders in very late life—expected to double over the next twenty years.

Also, for some years now, as health care costs have spiraled ever upward, state governments, which license, strictly regulate, and pay for much of the care in nursing homes, have tried to contain the higher costs of long-term care by limiting the numbers of nursing home beds. In response to the resulting gap in care and housing, we have seen the ballooning growth of less regulated assisted living facilities. Nursing homes now house those with the most advanced disabilities; newly built assisted living facilities suffice for many who in the past would have lived in nursing homes but are now required to live longer on their own. This housing trend improves the efficiency of the health care system, but poses many practical and emotional problems for elders and their families by forcing another transition when health further fails.

> While visiting Mexico, we met a friend for lunch at a street café. His mother, a very quiet and proper American, was with him, and a young Mexican woman, her companion, sat nearby. It took a little while before we recognized that our friend's mother had dementia. Her son's solution to her care had been to buy an inexpensive house in Mexico, where he had always wanted to live, and to bring his mother to live with him there, hiring very affordable around-the-clock helpers for her. A single local family provided reasonably high-quality care and a more affordable solution when compared with U.S. institutional care costs that can run from $50,000 to $80,000 or more per person yearly.

> ————————

> The family was twice asked to remove Aunt Sophie from nursing homes because of her disruptive behavior, moaning and chanting all day and hours of the night that hadn't improved after many trials of

drugs. Then her family heard through friends about a Filipino family that took one frail elder at a time into their small home and provided care. After three weeks with these kind caregivers, Aunt Sophie had stopped her crying out. She lived with them for the remaining two years of her life. Her daughter and her family visited her with the same frequency, but with a lot more satisfaction and peace of mind. She was admitted to the hospital for the last few days of her life at the advice of the doctor who followed her care.

Unspoken Concerns

As you have seen at each station, our shared Late-Life journey requires that we open areas of communication that might previously have been off-limits. The social and psychological dynamic will vary from family to family. As I have noted, during the Station of Decline, medical professionals tend to become more distanced from the very old and thus are less available for guidance and the initiation of such communication. The challenge becomes, "Who among the Advocacy Team is most trusted and most appropriate to initiate these conversations?" Way back at the Station of Stability, families began to explore legal necessities such as wills and advance directives. Such anticipatory discussions rightly presume that both crises and decline will happen, though it is never easy to predict exactly when. With the passing of each station, as an increasing sense of interdependency and trust develops between an elder and his or her family, the balance of initiative shifts more toward family members, friends, and the community within the Circle of Concern.

The two most important unspoken concerns in the Station of Decline have to do with loss of identity and loss of personal dignity. Elders in decline rarely have the energy to express and defend their individuality. It may not even have occurred to them that a part of what is making their lives more emotionally difficult at this juncture is the treatment (tones of voice, condescending or overfamiliar terms of address, and even baby talk) by helpers that reduces them to "just another old person." This casual degradation is most likely to happen, of course, with relocations to other "homes." All the details of a particular life have fallen away into repeated daily rituals of caregiving and the brief conversations that institutional schedules allow. How much more lonely is the plight of those who have no family to teach the staff who their father was before his decline!

Feeling a loss of personal dignity may be more regularly, though indirectly, expressed. This follows on the loss of control that the elder feels and is made more acute by descent down the scale of ADLs. Losing driving privileges was distressing enough back at the Station of Compromise, but needing help with bathing or using the toilet from a family member or a hired stranger is more of a blow to personal dignity. Responding to and softening these losses by more open discussion, gentle humor, and strong advocacy falls to the elder's support group.

Decision-Making in Decline

At this stage of your elder's journey, an understanding of "remaining expected years of life" is vital for good and humane decision-making. As I mentioned, in the case of an older person with multiple diseases who develops cancer, the institution of chemotherapy, radiation therapy, or surgery for cancer may prove so taxing as to use up not only all the energy available for healing and quality of living but also time itself—perhaps as much as half or more of the expected remaining months or years left to him or her. For frail elders, medical treatments may actually be more detrimental than a slowly progressing disease. At this Station of Decline, demanding treatments have major long-term implications that practitioners of Fast Medicine may not appreciate. Older patients may not fully or effectively recover enough from a given therapy to remain independent or even comfortable.

> My actuary friend Sam had a bigger and bigger smile as he approached ninety years of age. A lifetime of work with statistics had taught him how misguided much thinking and decision-making are, particularly as he and his peers neared their statistical and real ends. "The term 'average life expectancy' should really be called 'the fifty-fifty bet,'" he chortled at his yearly exam. "Folks just don't understand that *average* means that half of us are going to get there alive, and the other half will be dead. Speaking as a lifelong optimist, I've liked my chances. But you doctors should 'fess up when you talk with patients."

Sam was urging us to appreciate how short any elder's average remaining length of life may actually be. This reality is important when families wrestle with the issue of relocation, and it is of vital concern for Slow Medicine's humane medical decision-making. The way ahead will always have some difficulties that compromise an elder's quality of life. Years of disability-free living will always come to an end. Every decision that changes or threatens the status quo—"my life as I enjoy it now"—deserves a lot of thought. If an elder can eke out another few months of feeling well and happy, those months or years represent a significant portion of the remaining years of his or her life. Just being in the unfortunate position of having to contemplate a decision about leaving a home or embarking on a demanding course of therapy for a worsening health problem usually signifies that *an elder is already a member of the less well half of his or her age group and will, as an individual, have a lower likelihood of living to the point of average life expectancy.*

Suddenly, the future looks shorter and less rosy than we had hoped. Do we trade the reality that we know (present living circumstances or present symptoms) for an unknown that may diminish the quality of remaining days? My sister supported a "summer trial" for our mother, which happily turned out to last for fifteen months. In contrast, facing a six-month average life expectancy if he left his active leukemia untreated, my elder patient, Keith, chose a rigorous course of chemotherapy, hoping for an extension of "an average of twelve months." As things played out, he spent a difficult four months in the hospital and the last seven months of his life in a nursing home. Some outcomes turn on luck, some on statistical likelihood. As my actuary friend said, assuming one will be average is not always a good bet.

Practical Tasks at the Station of Decline

TRAVELING WITH A PARENT ON THE PATH OF DECLINE

Balance Concerns for Physical Safety with Fairness in Risk-Taking

The Station of Decline must engage these two opposing values. Bad or difficult events will occur—they always do. For instance, nearly everybody who lives long enough will fall . . . and older people often don't share news of falls with their families. (Doctors who understand Slow Medicine will ask not "Have you fallen?" but rather "When was your last fall?") How heavily will you lean on the physical safety argument when your parents are willing to risk some things going wrong in order to hang on to life as they are living it? Can you (and everyone who will join the discussion after the next fall) agree on how you all will deal with guilt (and perhaps even shaming—"What do you mean, she's living alone? In her condition!") when the inevitable crisis comes along? Do you understand that your parent is just as likely—perhaps even more likely—to fall and have other crises in new and unfamiliar living circumstances? Families and neighbors will differ in their capacity to tolerate risks, but this issue always underlies discussions about planning during the Station of Decline. By bringing the physical safety issue out into the open early and exploring the pros and cons of risk-taking, you will be elevating this issue to the level of prominence it deserves and head off the divisive role it often plays when it is not addressed in advance. Try to keep in mind that security is emotional and psychological as well as physical, and trade-offs are often required.

Coping with the Uncertain Balance Between Quality of Life and Further Medical Treatments

As the sands run down the hourglass, it becomes more and more difficult to see with certainty what value new therapies offer to halt the downward slide. The insertion of a coronary artery stent was clearly the right thing to do two years ago, but now an artery is blocked again. Is Mother really a suitable candidate now to subject to the stresses of another hospital admission and procedure? Would she do better if we simply provided support and tried to manipulate medications at home? Is the offered therapy more taxing than doing nothing? From Mother's point of view, where does the greatest quality of remaining life reside? It is so difficult in later stages of decline to ascertain the difference between the worsening of a known problem and the slow, up-and-down slide into diminished wellness and functioning that aging brings on its own. Uncertainties abound. And many choices can be truly evaluated only in retrospect.

Every new acute illness that comes along for an elder in Late Life has a high potential to become a chronic problem. An abnormal heart rhythm gets corrected to normal, the anemia gets treated to better "numbers," but the fatigue never fully goes away, and your parent's capacities continue to diminish. Success from a doctor's disease-focused perspective no longer coincides so closely with your mother's own sense of recovery.

Try to Elicit Feelings

The aftermath of the Station of Crisis brought sudden feelings of demoralization as everyone's emotional reserves ran down. In the Station of Decline, you can expect that some periods of *dispiritedness* become chronic for an elder. "I can carry on, but the effort leaves me feeling pretty low by the end of the day." The spirit starts out willing, but the body is not able. This condition is characteristic of life at this station and very different from depression. Our culture's overeagerness to fix "lows" with medications can greatly confuse an elder's mental and physical situation. I recommend, instead, caring attention, audible expressions of concern, and empathetic understanding. Be a good listener, and try to elicit an elder's feelings—their expression alone is often therapeutic . . . at least temporarily, which is all that may be possible.

Keep an Eye Out for "Failure to Thrive"

Frailty advances slowly, usually over years, and seldom catches family and caregivers off guard. Occasionally, however, a rapidly accelerating version of frailty that is termed *failure to thrive* catches hold, bringing a greater sense of foreboding and perhaps impending death. Often after some acute crisis, as though an internal switch were thrown, an elder's appetite and metabolism change. A kind of physical dissolution sets in. In these situations, diagnostic tests seldom turn up a cause, and all the medical and technical approaches we know are limited in effect. In an effort to break the spell, make the elder the absolute center of attention. This is the time for family and friends to gather close and bring all the emotional and spiritual support that can be mustered to attempt to reverse the downhill course.

Tolerating the Stresses of Chronic Care

If it hasn't already happened, there will be throughout this Station of Decline pressure to move a parent into an assisted living facility or nursing home. Increasing nighttime work deprives caregivers of adequate rest. Difficulty in providing personal care for an elder's progressive incontinence is a wearying strain. Then there is the mounting stress of managing difficult behaviors associated with dementia. The capacity to tolerate day-in and day-out stresses may wax and wane for caregivers, making it difficult to confidently say a situation is going downhill. One day the inevitability of collapse seems so clear; the next day both caregiver and elder rally to some degree. Family members are both spectators and participants in this process. As with all issues of stress, a fresh infusion of hands and support can offset the problem, at least for a while. See if you can persist for another month. Every one counts for your parent. Try to resist rash and sudden changes. Let decision-making play out very slowly. Seek out community support groups if you haven't done so already.

Consider All the Long-Term Care Options Now Available

In some places, nursing home design and care programs are being revitalized by innovations such as the "green house" movement to make institutional long-term care more homelike. Assisted living facilities and day care programs for elders and the disabled are springing up in every community. Just as our culture has shifted its views about having to be an inpatient in a hospital in order to get high-level technical care (now commonly available on an outpatient basis), so we are beginning to see that types of care—particularly for elders with dementia—that previously were provided only in nursing homes are equally well provided in more agreeable homelike settings. Some of the improved features are "country kitchen" common areas, fewer long hallways, fancier decor, and brighter lighting: in a word, these are less "institutional." Search your region for various innovative programs to get ideas on how they design for frailty and what their successes have been. This is where the cutting edge of better care is on display. And finally, while considering long-term care and evaluating specifically what each institutional setting can offer, consider once again how those services could be provided alternatively (and perhaps less expensively) while keeping your parent at home a bit longer.

Look into PACE

Just when the tide of nursing home growth was running high and extending into every community in the 1980s, along came a program out of San Francisco's Chinatown that showed a new direction for elder care. PACE (Program of All Inclusive Care for the Elderly) emphasizes stay-at-home living by supporting families with transportation, social services, day care, and personalized medical care delivered by the PACE geriatric team. Think of it as an *extensive* care unit—Slow Medicine's way of keeping an elder out of the hospital ICU. Our federal government's Medicare and Medicaid programs are actively promoting the expansion of this model throughout the country. PACE offers care-for-a-lifetime for selected elders who might otherwise have to live in nursing homes. Family satisfaction has been very high (www.npaon line.org). Other programs are copying aspects of this innovative model.

Consider Care Managers

Middle management has come to elder care. For modest to expensive hourly rates you can hire someone to oversee an elder's care and supplement your personal attending and direction. For many busy and distantly separated families, a care manager becomes a godsend. For other families, it is simply out of the question financially or proves to be just another layer of coordination and worry. Medical care systems that have experimented with the provision of care management remain somewhat divided about the ultimate value of these services. In our fragmented medical system, experienced care managers can organize tasks and save time gathering information, but don't count on them completely for the critical analysis of your parent's needs or sensitive monitoring of serious, evolving health issues. Evaluators of care management recognize that the skills involved can be acquired (and usually are acquired, perhaps more painstakingly) by actively involved family members. As a long-term investment, having a family member fill this role may make more sense.

Keep Track of Medical Records

Who knows what? Who is talking to whom? What if the doctors (and other health care professionals) are not talking to one another directly? Your elder's medical record is vital for properly coordinated care. Keep in mind not only that a person's medical records are being kept for the benefit of the patient, but also that the patient is the rightful owner of the record and its information. Does your parent—or do you—have any sense of what that record says about his or her current situation? Would it be helpful for the family to know more of what is written there? Will it be your responsibility to convey an overview of that record if there is a failure of communication between the different locations of your parent's health care? Or if there is an uninformed substitute physician on call?

Just as you advised your mother to use the emergency information packet in her home, so you need to keep copies or summaries of records on hand to provide better continuity and coordination of care. As you observe how the system works (or doesn't work), decide whether you need to step up your involvement by being included in the communication of this information. Is it time for your parent to empower you formally to have this role? You don't want to be caught peeking at records if you haven't cleared the right to do so. It is entirely legitimate to bring the issue of shared information into the open at the doctor's office, the nursing home, or the hospital.

THE NEXT LEVEL OF PREPAREDNESS

Learn to Practice "Watchful Waiting"

A common pattern of the Station of Decline is repeating bouts with a known chronic condition that lead to predictable "cycling" of the patient back and forth from home or a nursing home to the emergency room or into the hospital. Perhaps the problem is recurrent episodes of fast heart rate, shortness of breath (sudden anxiety or lungs closing down), or times when Mother is "not herself." If you are not careful, each occasion can be turned into a mini-crisis by anxious attendants. Even though you have lived through these crises before, an attitude of "I don't want this to go wrong on my watch" often spins elder, family, facility staff, and doctor-on-call off into urgent thoughts of needing to "do something." Resist these impulses. Let family, helpers, doctors, and institutions know how long you would prefer to have careful monitoring, personal attendance, and "watchful waiting" rather than a rushed judgment to evacuate Mother to the hospital yet again.

Since staff turnover, particularly in nursing homes, is common, you may have to repeat these conversations regularly. Above all, before you commit her to an ambulance ride, ask to be put on the telephone with your mother right then and hear for yourself that she is not in extremis. In dealing with a nursing home, ask that she be evaluated by the most experienced person readily available and keep talking to that person. Your parent and her attendants need your help and support. Chances are good at this station that most reruns will have the same outcome as the original episode. Prepare for these upsets in advance by having a family plan for twenty-four-hour, seven-day-a-week telephone availability.

See Adaptation as the Primary Goal

Your mother is having to adapt to accelerating losses, having to accept assistance, and coping with new and unfamiliar people, not to mention the daily reminders that life is draining out of the tank. In fact, adaptation is everyone's work at the Station of Decline. We must learn to deal with our own increasing uncertainties and anxieties about how best to respond; get through recurrent feelings of helplessness; resist temptations to deny or avoid what is going on; mute surges of anger; and cope with the consequent stresses forced upon us by our own busy lives—all this going on perhaps for years. We may often find ourselves resisting and resenting the difficult work of this station. An important part of continuing to care effectively for your parent is admitting the undersides of your own emotional reactions. If you don't explore these feelings regularly, sooner or later they will intrude into the lives of everyone. If you don't choose to join a support group or go for individual counseling, be sure to confide in friends who have experienced this difficult stage of life with a parent.

Recognize the "One-Way Street"

In our younger years we changed jobs, places of residence, and relationships with the understanding that these transitions could be accommodated, worked through, or rebounded from over time. In the Station of Decline, transitions for elders are usually irreversible. Parent and family alike run out of energy and perhaps courage. Rarely do an elder and family return to a previous living situation after a trial in institutional living. Elders know the odds in their guts; families may try to rationalize that these are only temporary arrangements. Before such a move, an open-ended and generous period of contemplation and exploration will serve you well. Learn about the successes and failures of friends and other families. Listen to everyone. Delay a decision for three months. Then start another round of discussion. Your search for instructive stories will prepare for the time when you all may actually be ready for that transition.

Learn About "Active Listening"

Developers of new medical technologies have their sights set on selling video monitors for the homes of elders for the sake of their adult children. But less intrusive and costly than installing video monitoring of your parent's apartment could be your own voice monitoring of his or her well-being through a daily telephone call. Studies confirm what we all knew: subtle changes from day to day in your parent's tone, voice strength, and inflections (those undertones you learned to read as a child and perfected an understanding of during adolescence) give you the real dope on what's going on. "Low spirits," "bad days," "loneliness," and even the early onset of illness can be detected by an experienced family member or friend before the train goes off the tracks—and certainly before even an experienced health professional might recognize any warning sign for problems ahead. If you're not good at this, think about attending a local course on "active listening." (It may help you with your siblings, too.) No one can be a bigger expert on a parent's voice than a former teenager trained in the same household.

Finding the Right Words

How do we find the right words to talk about losses that are naturally a source of pain for all? How shall we balance our talk about a future that will end in death with talk about fully living in the present? "What are the words that you will agree to let me use?" "If that term is difficult for you, Dad, tell me what I might say instead?" "Can we talk about future planning in a way that both of us find comfortable?" "How can we work together to make your wishes for you (and your wishes for us) come true?"

Although some spoken acknowledgment of "where things stand" may be useful for everyone's understanding, in my experience rarely does repeatedly dwelling on death, dying, and final advance directives prove satisfying for anyone. Our parents may not be as accustomed to ventilating feelings as we are and may even experience some shame in doing so. Expressions of love, conversations, and activities in the here and now are much more likely to promote meaningful interactions. Trust builds through shared decision-making, time spent together holding hands, singing, reading aloud, and other joint activities more often than through discussions of "what might be." Never underestimate the power of nonverbal communication. Our deepest emotional messages often are conveyed through the comfort of silence.

Update the Advance Directives

As frailty of an elder's mind and body sets in, illness will commonly tip your parent's situation from "competent decision-maker" to "compromised decision-maker." In the Station of Decline, your parent will find it harder to grasp issues, to reason, and to make good decisions. Have you discussed with your parent's doctor (and those who would be his or her advocates) just how decisions will be made if anyone senses that your parent has *marginally* lost the ability to make consistently good choices? Who will judge this, and how will it be judged? This issue often becomes a gray zone during an illness and, without advance thought and preparation, dominant personalities may come to overrule the best-made plans. Develop a consensus and solidarity among family members and those in the Circle of Concern. Now is the time for these discussions to begin.

Listen for Your Parent's "Life Review"

Ever since Dame Cecily Saunders launched the hospice movement and Elisabeth Kübler-Ross wrote *On Death and Dying,* the process of approaching death has been carefully analyzed. An important part of a person's "settling up" is to see one's life from the perspective of its completion. In the clinical world of hospice, this is called "life review," and it involves the dying person's telling important personal life stories. My understanding of the importance of this concept has greatly helped my own active listening at the bedside and in the examining room for all elders, not only those near death.

So when your parent starts telling you the story of his or her life or the details of illnesses, try to listen carefully and with interest, even if you've heard the narrative many times before. Particularly at the Station of Decline, when memories more frequently arise from the quiet pool of time that each day represents, every personal encounter has elements of life review in it. This recounting is not necessarily purposeful, but try to appreciate the enormous benefit of the comfort of feeling fully understood that it leaves with your loved one. Breathe slowly in and out (practicing your own Slow Medicine) and invite a new curiosity about what you are being told. Most stories can expand and deepen with a little prompting and genuinely interested questions about context. And even though you will hear the same stories tomorrow, there will come a day when you will be thankful you listened well.

Learn to Forget the Numbers

An understanding of how your parent is doing is seldom conveyed effectively by mere numbers. Unlike stories and images, numbers exclude "what it feels like" to be alive. Don't tell me my mother's weight this week or her blood pressure numbers today or what percentage of most meals she eats. Tell me about the best and worst things that happened to her this past week or month, and I will better understand her current state of being. Hearing about her one group outing and Happy Meal souvenirs alongside the lengthening naps that interfere with her eating tells me a much fuller tale. Politely listen to the numbers if you must, then solicit some stories if you really want to be in the know.

Learn How to Reduce Anxiety

There is no question that the Station of Decline is fraught with anxiety for everyone. It could be anxiety in response to the return of discomforting symptoms. Or it could be the anxiety that floated into your parent's consciousness one day for reasons that can't be articulated. ("I just don't know why I'm feeling this way.") Is it a foreboding of another impending betrayal by an aging body? Or random passing confusion? Or perhaps some sense that a dark cloud hovers overhead and the game of life is almost over? What can you offer to help bring an elder back from the stress of such moments? For example, for elders with breathing problems, calming and relaxing techniques and an open window and fresh air can relieve symptoms of breathlessness sometimes just as well as extra inhalations of medication or turning up the oxygen level. Nothing accelerates emergencies faster than an elder's anxiety about losing personal control or seeing confidence lost by attendants. Hang in there in a calming way until the first wave of panic passes. Remember what you learned in the Station of Crisis about nearness, calming touch, and soothing words. Don't get caught in the spiral of anxiety, especially from a distance.

Shift Your Focus from Cognition to Behavior When Dealing with Dementia

"It's not what you know or explain, it's what you do" that makes the difference in addressing the many daily crises—minor and major—of persons with dementia. Train yourself to respond to the mysterious, many-faceted losses of dementia by redirecting attention from whatever the source of discomfort or aggravation may have been. Point out what's happening outside the window or just outside the doorway. Ask your mother to walk to the kitchen and help you with some cleaning. Sit down with an arm around her and bring out the book of old photographs you've put together. Memories of the last upset often evaporate in minutes. Don't even try to understand what just happened; *unpredictability is a predictable part of dementia.*

BUILD YOUR ADVOCACY TEAM

Recognize and Promote Covenants

Personal loyalty and the unspoken covenant to remain engaged are two enduring gifts to an elder in decline. When "all has been done that can be done," your commitment to supporting a relationship to the end remains. Certainly there will be exceptions as helpers come and go and family members attend to other important matters. But nothing is more dispiriting to an elder and a circle of caregivers than to face growing isolation or abandonment. Now is the time consciously and formally to reenlist all members of the family. Although the conditions of renewed support may have to change, be sure to acknowledge the contributions everyone has made—including your own—and to ask sympathetically for their continued involvement. Not only does recruiting or replacing Advocacy Team members take time and energy, but every time continuity is interrupted, there is also a loss of understanding of the person—a foundation of Slow Medicine. A new doctor seldom achieves the same depth of connection with the elder in decline; new friends for your parents are hard to make if old ones depart. Attending to and celebrating your team every now and then are both necessary and well-deserved.

Solve Problems with Employers and Colleagues

The stresses of chronic care usually ripple out from the focus of your family concern into your community and your work. You may need to devote new attention to your employer and colleagues at work. Let us assume that during your parent's latest crisis, everyone at work was sympathetic and supportive. You needed to leave and be with him or her. Your employer and your fellow employees were relieved that your parent made it out of the hospital and expressed admiration for your committed engagement. Personal leave days covered your time away, and everyone pulled together to take up the work burdens at the job. However, additional time away (another visit to follow up and keep abreast of your parent's changing needs) may be more difficult for your work partners to absorb. Some will continue to sympathize and offer support. Other colleagues may have their own very different personal and family responsibilities to shoulder and, understandably, face more difficulty covering and making up for your absences.

Transformation of work around the burdens of elder caregiving is only slowly emerging as an issue in most workplace settings. Being wise early to the fact that the aged population is growing and that increases in elders' numbers and longevity are going to affect more and more workers in their forties, fifties, and sixties puts you in a vanguard position. Elder care is rapidly joining child care and flexible work from home as important issues for the twenty-first century. If these burdens are viewed as only individual and quietly shunted to the side to be worked out informally, broad support may well come more haphazardly and slowly. Use your personal story to help open your workplace to an exploration of how you will support one another when needs for caring arise.

Understand and Support Your Parent's Circle of Concern

Retirement has been viewed as a period for recreation, travel, and activities that enhance health and personal satisfaction. This was true for a newly retired nurse who soon confessed, "All of our neighbors needed so much help, we had no time for ourselves." Yet, in most communities, our elders rally to help one another with a dedication that other generations may only hope to achieve. "We are propelled into caring relationships—this is what we do at this stage of our lives," an older friend assured me.

As your parent's needs increase and individuals in the Circle of Concern step up to help you with support and care, spend some time learning what this means for these important folks in your parent's life. What stories propel them to step forward? What do they find satisfying? What wears them out? Many of these important, caring friends and acquaintances will remain in your elder's life through years of declining health. You have a chance here not only to appreciate and support them, but also to be enriched yourself by their values and ways of living.

Resist Withdrawing When Things Are Stable

You have worked hard and thoughtfully to create a living situation for your mother as she drifts down the river of slow decline. It can be so easy at the latter parts of this station to withdraw for some deserved rest. But don't let your withdrawal become chronic. In addition to being prepared to respond to sudden bad things that happen—the next crisis—how can you put your energies into some more positive affirmation of her survival? Keeping Mother's presence in your life and in the lives of others on the advocacy team takes some attending. During this long drift in decline, people tend to slip out of touch. Your own busy life asserts itself. Is some archivist in your family still generating stories, recordings, and images from the world your parent lives in, the life and rich history she still has for others to share? Can you bring a hymnbook to pore through with her that brings back memories? How does she respond when grandchildren or great-grandchildren bring in dolls or toys to show? Are there some new stories that have begun to come out during this time of life review that need recording? Have you actually written down family names and dates that you will want to know later? After years of hard work riding out crises, it is all too easy to let an institutional "autopilot" take over, leaving your parent, you, and others without enduring human connection. Patience, loyalty, and simply showing up are not showy virtues, but they can be far more sustaining than flashy rescues.

Make Caregivers Part of the Surrogate Family

As your elder's contingent of caregivers expands, you are creating a surrogate family. Depending on the length of time an elder stays at the Station of Decline and on the immediacy and intensity of the family's and friend's involvement, this surrogate family can be powerful and significant but sometimes difficult. Just as you experienced differences of opinion and values among siblings and in-laws around questions of what is best, so your elder's new surrogate family of caregivers will incubate their own opinions. It is easy to make the mistake of trying to ignore their views or override them as irrelevant. These attendants spend a great deal of time with your parent each day. Don't be surprised when strong responses and feelings emerge during periods of stress or change. Be observant and careful to note unarticulated attitudes and unexpressed feelings. Hidden currents can undermine your hard work. Properly done, your job has the additional responsibility of paying attention to the caregivers. This is true even when your parent is in the nursing home. Stay in touch. Show your concern and appreciation, especially during periods of changing health or illness. Something as simple as flowers or a jar of jam for the staff lets them know you care about them, too. It may mean more work for you, but you may feel more welcomed for recognizing that your parent's good care depends on all of you working together.

ENGAGE MEDICAL CARE

Practice Family Surveillance

Did the following issues get discussed and documented when Mother entered an extended care program?

- All of your mother's many medical diagnoses, which by this time may number a dozen or more.
- Doctors' attempts at predicting your mother's course (prognoses) and their degrees of accuracy.
- Present and past medications and their effectiveness; also, which medications haven't been evaluated or thought about deeply enough.
- All the cognitive and behavior impairments your mother has shown and how they have waxed, waned, or progressed over time, and what seems to bring them on or diminish them.
- A complete list of your mother's previous doctors (including all specialists) and how they can be reached if they are needed for consultation. Significant summaries of their findings might actually be collected for future reference.

Gather your family and members of your mother's advocacy team and brainstorm your core understanding of her situation to share with the staff. Although there are widely used "intake tools," such as the Minimal Data Set (MDS), that standardize information for all new nursing home enrollees, *your job is to particularize understanding.* Despite the vast number of forms (my mother signed nineteen when she first entered a nursing home—and she wasn't feeling well to begin with), don't count on institutional systems to convey what you more fully and particularly understand. Be polite and persistent and expect some resistance, since you will be bringing more paperwork to the staff, and they already feel overwhelmed. It is up to you to bring your parent's story to light. Support the staff's hard work and nurture these relationships. Before long they will begin to see you as a help, not a hindrance, and your parent as a person with a remarkable history.

Stay Connected to Your Parent's Doctor

Here resides an extraordinary and difficult dilemma for which you need to understand the background: very few doctors work in settings where care in the Station of Decline takes place. House calls have all but disappeared. Seventy-five percent of physicians spend no time and only three percent spend substantial time in nursing homes. Your mother may be one of the lucky ones whose doctor will still "attend" to her in this new setting; more likely she will face a new doctor—and a busy one at that. You will learn to appreciate what the nursing staff has struggled with forever: how to engage the doctor enough and in the right way. The nursing staff and your family want for your mother both routine attention and, when needed, rapid urgent attention from the doctor. But the doctor's response needs to be at a level of intensity that suits your parent and your long-crafted plan for *appropriate* Slow Medicine care. On the one hand, you may find yourself begging for some attention, and, on the other, you may be fending off a knee-jerk response that will have her packed into an ambulance and heading to the hospital emergency room for every problem. Your mother will not be able to manage this situation on her own. Only your regular involvement (which, even at the nursing home, includes attempting to anticipate crises) will keep everyone on the same page and help meet the challenge of changing health and needs.

The Role of Medications for the Patient in Decline

The medical profession's tendency toward "poly-pharmacy," the use of too many drugs, is risky for every elder. You should also worry about all those over-the-counter pills your parent has rattling about in the medicine cabinet, on the bedside dresser, on the kitchen table, and in the bag with other medications no longer used, but not thrown away. Hazards increase year by year from unsupervised medication-taking at home, ranging from misread labels (too small print, poorly understood directions) through interactions between drugs and with foods. Even if your parent relocates to an institutional setting, don't count on these risks disappearing. Poly-pharmacy is also a big problem in nursing homes.

An example of the complexity of decisions regarding medication for elders involves the risk of falling. *Every study done on falls in Late Life ties this risk to the number of medications being used.* Yet, despite long-standing evidence about the connection between drugs and falls, many doctors still hesitate to reduce an elder's medications.

Overtreatment for high blood pressure can result in falls and strokes brought on by too low blood pressure, often a bigger risk for frail elders. There is a long-standing international debate over the value of aggressively using multiple medications to lower blood pressure in Late Life. Earlier in life, preventing future damage makes clear sense. However, putting an elder at risk of more side effects (fainting, falls, confusion) for only a small theoretical reduction in stroke risk may not make sense. Geriatricians often find value in reducing or eliminating medications for elders for trial periods in the Station of Decline. Many patients simply feel better when they use fewer medications. Have a discussion with your parent's primary physician about the pros and cons of each and every prescription.

Bring Your Views and Push for Medical Consensus on "What's Going Wrong"

Over time, we become aware that Dad's recurring heart failure has taken its place among a host of other advancing problems. Now we also need regular input from kidney, lung, and psychiatry specialists. Each physician impresses us with depth of knowledge in his or her respective field, but in the end it falls to us to determine from observation and experience which of Dad's multiple problems might on any day be edging ahead. New therapeutic routines, new cautions, and new—and possibly interacting—medications make it difficult to determine exact reasons for Dad's continuing decline. Talk with his physicians about your views and ask that they *try together* to achieve consensus on what needs to be focused on most of all.

Latch On to a Nurse-Practitioner or Physician Assistant

The nurse-practitioner (NP) is everyone's darling in elder care programs at the moment and with very good reason. The perfect combination of "a doctor with time" and "a nurse with enhanced clinical skills," these women and men are being hired by elder care programs and physician practices in ever-increasing numbers. Find out if an NP or physician assistant (PA) might be available, get to know something about how these health professionals work, and sign your parent into the program. Lobby on behalf of these important clinical care providers so that their availability doesn't fall prey to the same pressures that are driving doctors away from patients' homes, assisted living facilities, and nursing homes. Your parent will benefit from their capable care.

Taking Stock

Decline requires endurance, for your parent, for you, and for your family. This long stretch of time brews a wide range of feelings, from discouragement and depression through fear and anger. "Do we have it in us to go through this?" you may find yourself asking time and again. For the most part the problems and situations you face are characteristically unchanging. Your parent's life has now become more static; the intensity of your own life remains high, separating you further from the daily life led by your parent. Yet there remains a strong connection. When tension strikes any part of the family—relationships, work, finances—the issue must now be seen in the light of how we deal with Mother or Father. Your fears arise around the question of what more your parent will need and whether those needs could be met without moving him or her to another location, something we are mostly trying to avoid. "Please don't let her get any worse, or we'll have to find another place and start all over again." The pressure to make decisions is shifting more and more to you as the adult child. Personal projection becomes a larger part of choosing among alternatives. "How would I want this done if it were me? How does it fit with my parent's wishes expressed in his or her living will?" Most of the small daily choices you must make are not likely to be covered by formal directives. More issues reside between the lines and are debatable. "Should we continue to ask the staff to help her walk when she really doesn't want to?"

Your parent's unhappiness and recurrent small crises can make you become critical of the health professionals and other caregivers, including family members, who direct his or her course and care. You may want to see your parent's failing as their failings, giving rise to anger and conflict about getting needs met. "If only she could have a busier schedule, more attention, a different sleeping medication, her life would be improved."

Guilt arises from opposing pressures, from your feeling of failure in preventing your parent's decline and the opposing readiness to simply let decline happen, "there being no other way." "Have we done enough?" "Should we get another second opinion?" "Do we have an effective medical advocate?" "Is it good enough not to send her to the hospital for another X-ray—it was so difficult for her after her last fall?"

And underlying it all is sadness, which weighs on you daily as you see your parent's life become more constricted, foreshadowing the inevitability of what's to come.

Prelude to Dying

———⊗⊗⊗———

"I sense a change in her spirit."
—NURSE IN LONG-TERM CARE

Again, a telephone call. "She was found on the bathroom floor,"
my sister Maureen reports. "She seems to be all right, but when I
was there at Christmas I thought she was failing much more." We
have shared this conversation a number of times—Maureen's growing anxiety countered by my denial (usually cloaked in "doctor
talk"). What really signals the beginning of the end? Bertha's interest in the world has contracted well inside the immediacy of her
surroundings. Her hours of sleeping, day and night, continue to
lengthen. She no longer initiates telephone calls or outings. She's
become a "responder." Emotionally, she is very at ease with herself,
laughing off things when they go wrong, including her "slow slide"
to the floor. "One leg wanted to go in one direction and the other in
the opposite," she chuckles when I call to see how she is doing. For
Bertha, this new-spoken lightheartedness has announced her acceptance of what is to come. Chair-, bed-, and wheelchair-bound,
she has shifted beyond "decline."

Having watched closely for some years, families learn to note the smallest and most subtle changes in the way a parent responds to the winds that regularly buffet his or her passage. As Mother's outlook changes with the illnesses and frailty that advance decline, they also see that her "craft"—the physical body she inhabits—has lost more and more of its seaworthiness.

The Station of Prelude to Dying can involve much uncertainty (rather like "one leg wanted to go in one direction and the other in the opposite"), almost to the point of your questioning whether your intuition is true. "Could she really be dying?" "Should I visit sooner?" Turning the corner toward dying doesn't mean that death is right around the corner. All the same, a noticeable shift toward separation from life often appears late in the Station of Decline and heralds the entrance, perhaps only transiently at first, to this next station.

All four siblings, none younger than eighty-five, were "holding on" near Terrell Point at the north end of Carriacou's small island. Now, one was reported sick—the youngest brother, "not right in the head," a wanderer with dementia. The other three tended him and the garden that was their main source of food with the exception of a few gifts now and again from neighbors.

When I got there, Lyman was indeed sick, breathing rapidly and laboriously, sweat beading on his face. An exam suggested pneumonia, perhaps complicated by heart failure. His brother and sisters were gathered near the bed and thanked me for coming. I offered to have the pharmacist drive out from the hospital with some medicines. "Maybe he will respond."

"Doctor, he's had a good life, and now there is no hope," stated the elder sister, declining the medicine and looking to the others for confirmation. "You came and did your best for him, and we thank you." Island culture and government policy encouraged "attended" deaths. The quiet in which we all then stood helped me to understand that it was time.

Acknowledging that death is near and achieving comfort in the face of this reality are challenges for those who are close to a beloved elder. How much of my view of this present downturn am I projecting onto my mother and her situation? At times, I wish for change—and the end—because of all the difficulties my mother faces from day to day. At other times, my burden of uncertainty about when something new and critical will happen to her seems more than I can bear. She has survived so many small crises. Sometimes, I am convinced that appropriate medical care has made a real difference for her. Other times, her survival seems fated to happen for reasons none of us can understand. How can she keep on surviving so many small strokes (or falls or acute bronchitis bouts or periods of withdrawal and poor eating)? Not only are we, as family and friends, amazed by her ability to endure, but even the doctors and nurses comment on how exceptional she is.

At this point in the Late-Life journey, there are many reasons for wishing for change from the status quo. Those who care for an elder directly are showing signs of tiring both emotionally and physically. Perhaps Mother will need a fresh team soon, with all the preparation and effort that requires. Financial burdens—caused directly by her care and indirectly by its impacts on you—are increasing. Frequently now, Mother talks about the "growing burden" that she perceives herself to be. "I never wanted to live this way," she adds.

As you watch and learn from stories of other elders and their families, you realize just how long these Late-Life journeys can last. You may find yourself reading obituaries in your local newspaper, noting how many people now live into their nineties. Does an obituary give any clues about where and for how long the last years of a diminished life were lived? Who in the family survived? Some children die before their parent—a tragedy for the elder, who would gladly have traded extended years in decline for the survival of an adult child. The reasons go on and on—all of us are deeply aware of real unfairness in life situations and of our growing willingness to embrace our own parent's separation from life.

Shown into a back room bright with sunshine, I stepped over a foot-high board barrier that minimally barricaded the door. A mattress on the floor, made with clean sheets and a quilt, held the diminutive figure, peacefully sleeping. Jeannie and I spoke softly together, and then I knelt on the floor beside the mattress to awaken her mother for the exam. Slowly roused, the frail old woman put her hands on my white, short-bearded face. *"Zut alors!* I am ready," she told the imagined figure she took me for, then closed her eyes, expecting heaven.

Let's review how our priorities and the practice of Slow Medicine are playing out. The great degree of differentness that each elder developed over long years of living is likely now to "disassemble" in equally complex, unpredictable ways. More and more now hinges on the person Mother is, and your best responses reflect your deepest understanding of her. During the Station of Prelude to Dying, diseases lose their relevance in both care plans and caring. Should we have expected anything else? Idiosyncrasies of character and physical constitution lead to particular vulnerabilities and illnesses, but that same process also leads to hidden pockets of strength. "His heart seems to go on and on, though the rest of his body has fallen apart." "Her strength of will got her through again." "Now I truly believe that faith makes a difference—day after day she shows such a serene acceptance of her plight." Individual differences are playing out.

Just showing up continues to be important. The loyal caring and continuing commitment of others allow an elder to find meaning in each day. By now you have probably bonded with the staff members who care directly for your parent and have figured out ways to show appreciation for their dedication. Ideally, your parent's new doctor has been with her long enough now so that personal affection has become a real and sustaining part of their relationship. Friends and family are fulfilling their covenantal roles. As Mother depends on all of us to sustain her, so her happiness or sadness each day has its effect on us. Even talk of seemingly inconsequential things has important positive consequences—just because it is faithful communication. Though there is nothing else that medications and other therapies can improve, if you have done your emotional work well, you and your parent will be reaping the rewards of your attachment.

> The early seventies swept him away from the limited surf of Cape Cod to the breakers of the Pacific. The youngest of four and the most estranged from their rigid, upright father, Richard, Al surprised no one in the family when he fled at seventeen, abandoning all contact except for an occasional note at Christmas. Now slowly dying from an untreatable liver cancer, Richard chose to move into a nursing home, where he felt his care could be better managed. Withdrawn, he asked that friends not come to see him, but he remained cordial to family visitors. The one other person he allowed in—at first reluctantly and later with enthusiasm—was Judy, the first-year medical student working with me on a several-month elective. Their talks, and particularly her listening, I believe, paved the way, although no one knew for sure why Al arrived when he did— after twenty-six years away. Generously welcomed by his siblings and mother, Al became the most loyal attendant for his father, at the bedside every day for the final month.

You are now in the station where you can expect to experience glimpses of a long life's end. It could happen at any time—a slight downturn in health spiraling into active dying. Still, more often than you can anticipate, the threat of death recedes yet again, only to return weeks or months later. Your loved one's boat swings in the wind, occasionally taking water over the gunwales. Death hovers nearby, and you hold your breath and pray—not necessarily for life or death, but for the "right thing to happen."

The Late-Life Condition of Aloneness

When I'm Alone

"When I'm Alone"—the words tripped off his tongue
As though to be alone is nothing strange.
"When I was young," he said; "when I was young . . ."
I thought of age, and loneliness, and change.
I thought how strange we grow when we're alone,·
And how unlike the selves that meet, and talk,
And blow the candles out, and say good night.
Alone . . . the word is life endured and known.
It is the stillness where our spirits walk
And all but inmost faith is overthrown.

—SIEGFRIED SASSOON (1886–1967)

Among so many other active concerns, we sometimes forget how alone an elder can be. By virtue of the way our culture is organized, many people suffer a social aloneness that isolates them from human contact. Aloneness may also come about because of the loss of a spouse or life partner, a daily experience of absence. Finally, there is the private, existential aloneness that comes with the settled emotional acceptance that our individual life will end, separating us from everyone and everything we have ever known.

Our culture's increased social aloneness over the past few decades has been well documented in sociological studies such as Robert Putnam's *Bowling Alone: The Collapse and Revival of American Community*. The sense of community that our parents and grandparents experienced during the Great Depression and World War II, and practiced thereafter in widely shared public activities, has given way to the isolating pressures of our modern economic mobility, broken marriages, scattered families, private transportation, and technologies of home entertainments. More and more Americans live in one-person households. Aging increasingly brings with it a kind of enforced separation along with a steady flow of losses through disability and the deaths of significant others. "Harry can't play golf any longer." "My old neighbor died in Ohio, where she went to live near her daughter." Few today would argue that we actually become less alone socially as we grow old, though there are countervailing programs. Elders in higher-density residential communities enjoy common dining and a variety of shared activities. Local programs (senior citizen centers, community exercise programs, transportation systems for the elderly, church activities) have been developed to offset social aloneness. Despite these strong efforts, the balance tilts toward increasing isolation for many, if not most, elders.

The isolation that comes from the loss of intimacy brings a different kind of loneliness. Close relationships decrease in number with aging. Distance and difficulty with travel make for less continuity. Many living situations, in fact, preclude the development of new intimates. Marriages and partnerships end through separation, illness, divorce, and death. Intergenerational interaction—grandparents to grandchildren and traditionally based on play, sharing, and active caregiving—is limited now by distance and infrequency of contact, often consisting only of telephone calls or e-mails. An older person's impaired hearing reduces his capacity to use the telephone with as much satisfaction. Modern technologies are beyond the understanding of many. Much less often now do elders actually sit in the presence of their families, sharing comfortable familiarity just by being together. "I only see them at Thanksgiving or Christmas." There is much less physical contact, too. Widows and widowers suffer from the tangible loss of daily human touch. "My friends and family have lives of their own. Why burden them with sharing mine?" Where does one search for and how does one latch on to intimacy in this fragmenting world?

The kind of loneliness that is existential may be less apparent to those of us who are younger and in the thick of our lives. This special, end-time aloneness, which deepens and moves forward on its own, comes with acknowledging that you will soon leave life as you know it. Perhaps younger adults ignore this experience of elders because it is the hardest to "fix." The emotional work of old age generally brings an acceptance of this pulling away from the world, a peaceful understanding of the unavoidable necessity of final separation.

An exploration of these emotional conditions (along with the loneliness and solitude that may come with them) is often neglected by health care professionals or family when other discussions of health, illness, and dying occur. These three dimensions of growing aloneness give an elder much time and opportunity to process his or her place in life's journey. A person's inner life is a privileged place for health professionals, friends, and family members to discover, difficult though that uncovering may be at times. Such exploration should be done with the deepest respect. In this intimate place, one should not be quick to judge the thoughts, attitudes, values, and preferences that are disclosed. Often, a deep vein of denial may mask and defend this quiet place near a person's center. Some elders may even make light of this aspect of their lives. Yet I have seen Slow Medicine's active bedside listening open the door to an elder's spiritual center.

When I first met him, his special gifts didn't leap out. A former businessman, Tony had struggled for years with advancing, and now severe, congestive heart failure. He was quiet and shared little of his personal life during his first several visits to my office. Then, he rather suddenly remarried and seemed quite happy. Indeed, his marriage coincided with the stabilizing of his heart failure. But soon another difficult period arrived: kidney failure with increasing weakness and need for care, and finally, a move to the nursing home. Attending him there, I first heard the stories from his nursing aides. Tony began to talk about his own life, but he was also a good listener. Even with his health deserting him, mostly confined to his room and too weak to do much physically, he both talked and listened. Through this generous impulse of sharing Tony came to be known and to know and support his helpers, in ways they hadn't experienced before. They shared with one another their intimate stories of struggle and difficulty with an attentiveness and gentleness that was mutually healing. Though he was dying, this final period of his living was rich. He simply attended to what was immediate to him through small conversations, but he both shared and paid attention so very well.

The understanding achieved through these various conditions of aloneness clarifies spiritual values by which older individuals operate in health and in illness. Particularly in advanced age or in crises where death may be near, an elder's acceptance of separation becomes our guidepost. Perhaps not consciously communicated, this compass of abiding personal truth must be sensitively sought. Even if elders cannot articulate their perspective fully (or, in some instances, at all), they will operate from it when facing decisions. These deeper responses to the human condition of aloneness, sadness, and loss reflect the summation of a life and are the substrate for the work of family, friends, and health professionals in the Station of the Prelude to Dying.

Isabelle showed up "yellow" in my office. I could see her subtle change of hue and noticed how her clothes hung more loosely on her. When she looked at me, I also knew that she knew. The clinical details don't matter as much at ninety-three years of age. The cancer was in her pancreas. She was experiencing little pain; perhaps she would call it "difficult indigestion." For the remaining eight months of her life, her "best medicine" was having her old calico cat curl up on her belly while she napped in sunlight on the couch. They would purr together there in shared comfort. Two weeks before her death, Isabelle asked to take some Tylenol. Her helpers supported her with increased hands-on care near the end, helping her to fulfill her wish to die at home.

Practical Tasks at the Station of Prelude to Dying

READY YOUR UNDERSTANDING

"Hypermaturity"

Old trees fascinate me. I have read about clubs formed to visit ancient trees just to be in their presence. Many specimens in my own neighborhood are majestic in their full maturity, and others are so gnarled and badly rotted I expect the next windstorm to take them away. Still, even hypermature and diseased trees can sprout a new, if very diminished, canopy of leaves, drawing up from the surrounding soil enough nutrients to survive another winter. Understanding hypermaturity comforts me in my work during the Station of Prelude to Dying, helping me to appreciate miracles of human endurance when the gift of continuing life is upheld by a person's remaining inner strengths and by the abiding love and benevolence of others.

Late Near-the-End Stages of Common Terminal Illnesses

Heart and Lungs

Expect problematic acute symptoms (breathlessness, anxiety) along with chronic fatigue and loss of appetite as organ failure plays out. Attending to rapidly waxing and waning symptoms can be very demanding for caregivers and may require numerous adjustments to medications undertaken with advice from doctors and nurses. With organ failures, expect small—and occasionally large—recurrent crises with difficult-to-control and therefore more frightening symptoms. People suffering from heart failure often die "sudden but expected" deaths after a series of lesser crises. At this station, comfort for patient, staff, and family comes from knowing that upsetting symptoms can still be alleviated. Set up communications with medical care providers that allow rapid responses but, for elders and families desiring comfort-oriented care, avoid as much as possible the stress and upset of transporting your elder elsewhere for care.

Strokes

Strokes present a very different picture from organ failure. Though they come and go, small stroke symptoms are usually less frightening for elders (who are often not conscious of their condition). Experienced caregivers learn to be less fearful and more tolerant of these recurrences. For larger (more damaging and longer-lasting) recurrent strokes, you will need to plan for your elder's interim support—at home, in the hospital, or in long-term care. At this Station of Prelude to Dying, most care for a stroke-burdened elder will be palliative, that is, focused on lessening discomforting symptoms.

Cancer

Cancer is known as a "wasting disease," but pain is the symptom most feared by those who suffer with it. Fortunately, clinical pain management is getting better and better. As much as actual physical pain, a person's fear of pain must also be promptly addressed. Acute crises are frequently associated with not "being on top of" a person's pain. Prevention of difficult-to-tolerate levels of pain—using medications, alternative or complementary therapies, and psychological and emotional support—must be a caregiver's priority. When the medical and nursing staff and supportive family and friends are fully engaged, there is almost always a way to establish a program that allows elders to find a place of comfort.

Mini-Crises

During this period of winding down, several other common recurring crises arise for frail and disabled elders. "She is simply not herself," report the caregivers who are with your mother day in and day out. It could be the start of an infection; it could simply be some waning of energy leading to a bad day. Often the cause is not clear in the beginning; many times it never becomes clear, even with thoughtful and appropriate attention to her situation. At this station, to help an elder through these transient mini-crises, we should promote responsible observation rather than premature (and perhaps unnecessary) medical intervention.

Fever is another symptom that arises and may herald a crisis. Often the simple response of getting the elder to drink more fluids solves the problem by correcting some minor dehydration or providing extra means necessary to fight a mild infection. This simple treatment also offers comfort. Though many doctors and nursing homes in these circumstances jump at once to insert a needle and "hang an IV," the more time-consuming, but safer and gentler, coaxing down of fluids serves most elders just as well and without the anxiety and discomfort.

Near deaths: "Something happened. We thought we were going to lose her. She seemed to go into a fade." A simple faint? A heart rhythm problem? Reaction to a medication? How many times does an elder at this very late station get within mere minutes of dying and then quietly come back? If your parent is in a health care facility, these flickering moments are more likely to be witnessed, and you will have to respond to these reports. On these occasions, your parent's advance directives backed by your direct involvement will guide everyone on how to proceed. In all such situations, staying in close touch over several hours by telephone or going by for an extra supportive visit is helpful to your parent and the attending staff. You may need to do this repeatedly.

GET PREPARED

Keep Mother Moving

Sometime back, we recognized that building muscle strength, flexibility, and stamina was no longer realistic for Mother. However, you can help to keep her going in little ways—a little time in a favorite chair, getting into and out of a wheelchair, shifting in bed to take a look at something you want to show her. All of these little motions improve circulation and alter pressure points on paper-thin skin. Help to stave off those problems that, once established, cause discomfort and suffering. Think of this practice as helping with your parent's body's "microsystems," providing skin protection and relieving little and big joint aches. Itchy or breaking-down skin, as well as aching shoulders, hips, and back, can be avoided by regular small changes in position. *Keep your parent moving. Find a soothing lotion. Give a little massage. Be a hands-on supporter.*

Let the Arts Enrich Days

Activities for elders in day care and residential care, including assisted living and nursing homes, are quite varied these days—group exercise, small crafts, music and singing, playing Bingo (my mother's favorite). Changes of routine are usually stimulating. However, as energy runs down in this Station of Prelude to Dying, in-bed, single-person activities may be all that your parent can manage. Larger and more formal activities may get neglected because of lack of time or sleeping schedule or seeming uninterest. Yet, listening to music, hearing the spoken word in brief stories and poems, looking at family albums, and holding and experiencing small treasures together can offer important shared experiences when conversation stales or fails. Engage this smaller sphere.

As you choose the stories, music, and objects that you want to share with your parent, consider what has value and meaning in your years together. This is a good time to share the important emotional and psychological touchstones of your own life. Don't miss this opportunity for intimacy. Read a poem or tell a story you love. Seek a middle ground—talk about topics beyond what was eaten for lunch but nearer to home than the difficult things going on in the larger world. Strive for "emotional immediacy" when making your choices.

Accept Chronic Uncertainty

As an adult in the prime of life, you take pride in managing your family, community, and work life with confidence. In a crisis, you reflexively turn to honed and tested skills to exert control and direct events. During the latter stations of life, however, chronic uncertainty and the irremediable nature of your elder's problems can make you feel very uncomfortable. The course of an elder's slide toward death is as uncharted as death itself. You can't eliminate all "near misses" or the anxiety that such episodes create (usually much more for you than for your parent). After working for so long to anticipate and forestall every emergent difficulty, you now face worsening anxieties about what might come along next and when. In these uncertain circumstances, many capable people respond by becoming hypercontrolling. At this end-time of the shared journey, learning to exercise more measured judgment and limited action has more merit. Uncertainty will prevail. *Your work now is to get yourself emotionally "centered."* Except for insisting on kindness, spend less energy trying to control the details of care.

Learning to Soften in the Presence of Death

Who can teach us to be comfortable with the limits of our powers and the idea of death? We know in our gut and in our hearts that we are on the brink of loss—Mother has in her own way given us that message. How do we learn to make room in our hearts for her passing? This is a time when the ancient social model of care offers us more than the modern medical model. Years ago, most doctors attended deaths with some regularity, achieving through repeated experience a comfort with the limits of their powers, and they conveyed this acceptance to families. Today, hospital doctors' encounters with death are usually brief and in circumstances of acute crises (often with an attendant sense of personal failure when death, not recovery, ensues).

In our society, people "dying chronically" are relocated outside hospitals to fade away over months or years in nursing homes or private home care. They are attended there by only a small minority of physicians or, more commonly, by nurses with little involvement by doctors. More and more now, families are left on their own to find practical guidance and emotional support through this time of loss. How can you gain comfort in the presence of impending death? Hospital chaplains, ministers, and hospice workers can lend support to you as well as to your dying elder. Ask others about their journeys to the mountaintop. Most people will welcome your interest. Retelling and sharing stories, you will find, can make this experience both more emotionally tolerable and humanly rich.

Improve Your Self-Care

For decades clinical observation and medical research have shown that the emotional and physical interplay of "stresses bearing down" and "support holding up" determines how people fare during times of chronic stress. You have already experienced how this works during your parent's journey: sometimes you cannot easily change your burdens, but you can change how you support yourself. Caregivers can easily get caught in a mind-set that perceives—often correctly—that if they retreat the least bit from their day-to-day duties, the fragile house of cards will fall. All their energy goes into making things work for an ailing loved one. Yet, failure to acknowledge and address one's own personal health and emotional needs usually means that over time the "support holding up" the caregiving will weaken. Then things fall apart even sooner, with sad results for everyone. Getting all who are involved with supporting a dying elder to submit a self-care plan at this station brings this critical need out into the open. Don't be cowed by those who dismiss this suggestion with a curt "I can't take time for myself with all I have to do." Talking about a self-care plan now may provide someone a chance to ask for help. Neglect of self now means a high likelihood of requiring more urgent help later.

Deciding About "When to Call the Family"

Not everyone can be at the bedside when a potentially terminal problem arises for your mother. How do you want to instruct those who are there to alert you to significant changes in her condition? Although nursing homes and other facilities certainly operate under regulations about "when to call family," there are always some judgments that are in the gray zone. How unrousable is she? For how long? How do you want these finer judgments to be shaded? Are you all in agreement? Both clinical uncertainty and human fallibility can lead to situations where someone gets upset about "not being appropriately informed." Can you help your caregiver sister or the nursing home staff by stating agreed-upon family preferences? These end-of-life situations can evolve at two extremes. An elder dies suddenly, and the family demands to know, "Why didn't someone call earlier?" Or, when the elder's sixth—or tenth—recurrent blackout is reported by telephone, the family is upset to be alerted, only to have "nothing happen" yet again.

Institute a Communication Tree

None of us can intuit accurately how more distant family and friends want to receive communications related to a failing elder. Start open discussions now about such matters with the extended family and the broader Circle of Concern. Construct a written list of who will call whom to pass on news and avoid hurt feelings. My wife learned of a dear aunt's sudden illness and death weeks after the funeral; her father, under the stress of circumstances, mistakenly thought he'd informed her. Communication trees spread the work and extend the process to include others in the telling of the story, itself of value during times of crisis and death.

Talk About Funerals, Burial Plots, Memorial Services

A lot of Late-Life planning should be behind you at this station. Presumably you have worked together through simple advance directives, learning along the way that these were not mere onetime declarations that got filed away somewhere, but an actual process that needed ongoing, even increasing attention and revision in order to help decision-making be truly reflective of your elder's evolving circumstances and values. Similarly, financial planning and wills were probably undertaken with less emotion and completed long ago. A few elders may have expressed preferences for their own funerals and memorial services, bought their burial plots or arranged cremation, and even written their own obituaries. You may be among the lucky families who have already raised these more emotional issues in a calm and timely fashion. More likely, you are one of the many now wondering how to break the ice for discussing these very practical concerns. Is the family ready for the feelings that will be generated? Who in the family will broach this subject first?

ENRICH YOUR ADVOCACY TEAM

Embrace Slow Medicine's Partners: Palliative Care and Hospice Care

There are some potentially wonderful allies to enrich your advocacy team as the horizon closes in for your parent. Who would not want "humanistic care" for your elder? Yet palliation and hospice care turn out to be some of the most emotionally and logistically awkward areas of health care to engage. Palliation, in its most straightforward form, is certainly part of what all of us desire when we are ill or injured, that is, close attention paid to relieve painful or discomforting symptoms and suffering. Paying attention to palliation doesn't mean giving up on continuing to address an underlying disease.

Increasingly, families of elders at this Late-Life station have begun to understand the value of turning to palliative or hospice care. Yet fear and denial keep vast numbers of elders and their families from engaging in this discussion in a timely way. An expanded advocacy team can facilitate your learning about the thoughtful, comforting, and effective enhancements of care that hospice brings. When elders can no longer easily judge or make decisions on their own, families and advocacy teams can build trust and comfort by presenting and endorsing options as a group. Those who opt for palliation and hospice care almost invariably report high satisfaction with care and better times for all during this difficult period ... and afterward often express a wish that they had engaged this help earlier.

ENGAGE MEDICAL CARE

Focus on Symptoms When Dealing with Medications

All along the Late-Life journey, you have learned that the best quality of care for elders is achieved by paying attention to individual needs and balancing those against recommended standard protocols. This is especially true in these last stations of Late Life. However, this vital element of Slow Medicine is greatly complicated by the fact that quality of care in hospitals and nursing homes is evaluated in part by protocol-defined "appropriate medication use." (If condition A is present, medication X should be used—always.) Anything short of that can result in a demerit. As I have said before, for elders very close to the end of life who end up in hospitals or for those who live in nursing homes, it is much less clear that standard protocols offer value and sustain quality of life. (For instance, at some point for an individual, continuing "preventive" blood-thinning medications may cause more crises than their discontinuation would.) At the same time, focusing on medications that relieve troublesome symptoms is invariably useful.

Geriatricians know that an elder's greater comfort and quality of days may actually be achieved by eliminating some medications, or at least reducing their use. There is no way to do this short of careful, regular evaluation, altering doses to see how an elder responds. As the body weakens, many medications that had been tolerated in the past begin to cause subtle side effects that actually diminish a person's quality of life—loss of appetite, mild nausea, sedation, confusion, physical weakness, sleeping difficulties. Encourage your parent's doctor to consider the need for possible changes—as opposed to the more common practice of routinely continuing medications forever. Appropriate adjustments may make your parent's final months less troubled by side effects of unneeded drugs, freeing him or her to be more responsive to the remaining pleasures of life.

And . . . there will always be another new drug to try—modern medicine regularly discovers a last-ditch treatment offering some small hope of improvement to those with advanced diseases. On rare occasions, all of us have seen an unusual suggestion work for a while. Coming from well-meaning friends, the lure at this station of "Hasn't she tried ____?" may be hard to resist. What so often gets neglected in the push for new interventions is the systematic use of already known and effective palliative treatments to relieve common symptoms of slow decline and dying. Simply relieving mild but persistent pain, constipation, anxiety, and itchy skin can dramatically improve a failing elder's daily life.

Become Familiar with POLST
(Physician Orders for Life-Sustaining Treatment)

Oregon has led the way in developing a system to improve the specificity, documentation, and implementation of advance directives in nursing homes. Studied and written about extensively and widely promoted, the POLST system goes beyond the usual general advance directives that concentrate on DNR orders familiar to anyone entering a hospital or nursing home. Expanding the discussion of important, and commonly faced, medical decisions for elders with advanced illnesses, the POLST approach addresses diagnostic testing, intravenous fluids, tube feeding, antibiotics, and transfer to the hospital. These medical interventions are commonly proposed to failing, frail, demented, and ill elders and their families. POLST encourages discussion of these options in advance of need. Get familiar with this expanded range of decisions before you need to make them.

Food and Drink: Let the Patient Be the Guide

We are naturally drawn to nurture our loved ones. The provision of food and drink has always been a caring response in times of difficulty. I consider the hand-feeding of a disabled, weakened, frail elder to be one of the greatest sustaining activities and expressions of care and love that we can offer. Providing an elder with nutrition by aiding eating (for many, one of the last remaining pleasures) is simply more caring and humane than "delivering" nutrition via tubes. At this late station in life, there will often come a time when an elder resists eating because it is more difficult to eat and drink than it is to forgo these activities. How then will we respond? It is hard to relinquish these most deeply ingrained expressions of love and support. In such circumstances, you may take some comfort from studies done on food and fluids at this end-of-life stage confirming what many clinicians have long noted: *a gradual falling off of intake (first of food and later of fluids) doesn't in fact create a crisis of discomfort for the patient.* At the same time, paying careful attention not to overlook a return of an elder's drive to eat and drink again must be a part of our continuing care. We should allow the individual to guide us in indicating his or her desires. During this Late-Life station, decreasing calories and fluid intake seldom leads to dramatic changes or a rapid demise. Think of those drying autumn leaves that continue to cling to the branches.

Who Will Respond to Crises . . . and How?

Being "wrong-footed" in sports can make elite athletes look clumsy. There is a high likelihood that any one of the following—caregivers' inexperience, failure to know the plan, new staff members, fatigue, fear, anxiety, outside pressures, midnight jitters, the dark shadow of a long night—could set off a series of events that will unbalance you, at least briefly. Despite all our best efforts to secure your parent a humane and peaceful "letting go," many moments can come along when someone or something provokes panic and uncertainty and questions your hard-won acceptance that death may come soon and naturally. Observe patterns of care for other dying elders. As with any chain, your supportive planning with and for your elders as they near the end of life is only as strong as the weakest link. A doctor on call who is unfamiliar with your parent's situation, a "traveling" (substitute) nurse, a staff jittery from having just recently managed a conflicted family crisis—any of these things and many more, all of them independent of your family and your parent, may necessitate more hard, emotional work by you and your advocacy team. At this station be sure to have your parent's advance directives in hand and review your "endgame" strategy with everyone regularly. Vigilance is still the order of the day.

Taking Stock

This is truly the "walking the walk" station. You can now count on the confidence you have gained through practicing Slow Medicine. You have come to know your parent more fully. This is the time of beginning to let go emotionally. Still, it is likely that your confidence in your deepest understanding of your parent and your guidance for him or her at this stage may be challenged. Conflict may occur between family members, within the larger advocacy team, and with more newly arrived health professionals. Not everyone comes to recognize your parent's subtle new communications about his or her wish to escape the burdens of daily living. Uncertainty, which has challenged your understanding all along the way, is overcome in an individual way. "I sensed last week in our conversation that she wasn't quite ready." Different messages may go out to different family members. A dying parent responds in different ways with different children. "I am so sad, because we are still like oil and water in our relationship," a dying ninety-four-year-old confided to me in reference to her middle daughter. For a period of time these differences between members of the near circle of care may seem insurmountable. You may need to go over the advance directives and review the decisions that your parent and you all have taken along the way again and again in an effort to achieve clarity and consensus. One of you may feel you are (or are labeled as) the "cold-hearted one." You may feel you are getting this same message from health professionals, who continue to express hope for some extension of better times ahead or who are uncomfortable with death themselves. Fear and anger may arise within, even for the best-prepared.

At the same time that you are wrestling with confidence in your deeper understanding, you may be feeling a growing peace in knowing that your parent and you are approaching the end of the journey. Gradually, as time passes and consensus comes to surround your parent, you may be increasingly able to accept this new reality. In anticipation, you can feel the emptiness ahead of you. Sadness reappears when you start actually making the plans—preparing to deal with a funeral home, to plan a memorial service, to find a cemetery plot to have in readiness, to discuss where ashes might be scattered or placed.

Spiritual tasks may present themselves. "How will I find sustenance and renewal for myself? Do I have a spiritual practice to turn to? Would it be good for Mother and me to pray together? Should I bring my own children into her presence more regularly now? How will we discuss death in my own family?"

You have caught a glimpse of the near future, but you are not yet there.

Almost a thousand years ago, a Tibetan named Milarepa
spoke words that every caregiver would do well to take to heart.
"Hasten slowly," he said, "that you may soon arrive."
Hasten slowly, as caregivers and care receivers,
  that you may reach the destination you each seek,
    and in the manner you each deserve.

Hasten slowly, and learn the practice of patience—
  patience with the person you care for,
    and patience with yourself.
Hasten slowly, and learn the art of forgiving,
  as you look into one another's eyes,
    and as you see your own face reflected there.
Hasten slowly, and learn the discipline of being sturdy enough to bend,
  and firm enough to yield.
As you do so, your caregiving will assume strength
  it would not otherwise have.

—JAMES E. MILLER, *The Caregiver's Book:*
Caring for Another; Caring for Yourself

Death

———∞∞∞———

"You'd better come now."
—HOSPICE NURSE

At ninety-two years old, Bertha assures us she is prepared for
death, although she has not yet looked death in the eye. Major
illnesses have taken their toll, and for short periods we feared the
worst, but the nurse's last call has not yet come. Our mother
remains more prepared for her death than we are. Or so I think,
until a telephone conversation one morning when she tells me
that she woke in the middle of the night "very scared" and the
feeling persisted. "Have you become afraid of dying?" I ask.
"I really don't think so," she responds, "but I feel very alone and
afraid." We talk for a long time, and when I call back a couple
of hours later to check on her, she says the feeling has passed.
It hasn't returned. In the months since, despite this one stretch
of fearful hours, the emotional burden has shifted back to us.
When will it happen? How will she actually do her dying?
Equally important, how will we do?

I have been at a person's bedside near the time of death hundreds of times and have attended the actual moment of death dozens of times. It is familiar to me as a doctor, but much less familiar as a son. I was with my grandfather very near to his death. I first stood over my father's (and his father's) grave when I discovered its location a mere decade ago. As with any family in similar circumstances, I am both prepared and unprepared. The tale is yet to be told.

Death in Late Life

By late life, most elders and their families—and certainly those taking care of them professionally—recognize that life must come to its natural end. Anyone who lives to a ripe old age is acquainted with death. In general, the longer the journey, the more comfortable our aged parents become with the idea of death. Family members have already passed away; friends are dying regularly. Although a few elders may be frightened at the imagined process of dying, many fewer fear death itself. This does not mean that they welcome death. Up to this point for most, life has remained far too important to choose the alternative.

But since the journey of Late Life for the majority of elders is now so long and so slow in its unfolding, we should not be surprised that much uncertainty remains about exactly when the time of death will arrive. I have witnessed situations where the readiness to die comes to an elder, but to no one around him or her. A family will hear, "I have lived too long" or "I am living too poorly." An elder rightly senses death's nearness while the family and friends faithfully hold out hope for more time. "Perhaps this is going to be another of those periods that he's gotten through in the past." Close caregivers and the professional staff do well not to argue. Eventually, elders and those who care for them at this culminating station reach a consensus that death is very near.

By being fully engaged through all the preceding stations of Late

Life, we have built the emotional and spiritual capital to support ourselves during the Station of Death. Our hard work and sacrifice have better prepared us for "closing the circle of life."

> With each small stroke, Joe was admitted again to the hospital for an exhausting stay. With each futile cycle, it became clearer that nothing could forestall his deteriorating course, and he knew it. The last was one hospitalization too many for him and his wife. When the doctors advised a feeding tube and relocation to a nursing home, Sally signed her beloved husband out against medical advice (AMA) and took him home to die.

Diverging Perspectives

Inevitably, problems of letting go will arise for family members and friends at a distance. In our world of geographically separated and often fragmented families, there will naturally be some individuals who enter the scene only close to the time of death. Even if communications have been regular and thorough, these later arrivals will not usually have the emotional advantages of caregivers, whose daily involvement with an elder has earned them a more settled understanding of where things stand. Under such circumstances, it may prove a major task to bring everyone to the point of accepting the inevitable. Often, the pain of impending loss is so great that late arrivers bring upset and conflict to the deathbed. You cannot expect their instant acceptance and easy incorporation of the extensive emotional work already done by long-standing caregivers and attendants.

On the other hand, it occasionally happens that friends and family members at some distance from the caregiving trenches can provide helpful perspectives on choices to be made, even acting as caring, neutral mediators when conflict arises.

Over the week their father was in the ICU, sustained by breathing and feeding tubes inserted at the time of emergency surgery, a divergence of opinion widened between the brother and sisters. The brother, himself a doctor, wanted to do everything medically possible to help their father survive. The sisters wanted to honor their father's expressed desire not to be kept alive by "heroic measures" only to be relegated to a nursing home. When feelings escalated to heated discussions over the eighty-nine-year-old patient's bed, the father's consulting cardiologist and personal friend of twenty years convened a family meeting. After calmly summarizing the contending views and asking if he had stated the issues correctly, the elder doctor confided that he and his wife (an old friend of the father's as well) had similarly conflicting views on how to proceed. He admitted that all the women were less afraid of death and more accepting of loss. The men, feeling discomfort with failure and bound by their professional training to act, were emotionally less accepting. They needed a little longer. Successfully negotiating a grace period of two more days, the family waited to see what time would bring. Soon, the father's kidney failure made everything plain. The tubes were removed, and he died within hours.

Trust and the "Good Death"

If there is one single element that underlies a good death (an expected, supported, well-attended death in a location of choice), it is trust and its impact on the spirit. Do the dying have family, friends, and health care professionals who are trusted to read their situation correctly? Do they feel that what is happening is natural, inevitable, and fully supported? These are the final gifts of comfort that loved ones can give. For this to happen, a lot of work must have taken place in advance—all those months and years of showing up through thick and thin, all the hard work of making arrangements and speaking up for your parent along the way, all the quiet support of just being near.

Walking cold into a situation of such emotional intensity and hoping to develop the trust necessary to provide a context for appropriate care are supreme challenges. Yet that is what many unprepared families and elders face. In circumstances of limited trust, all the difficulties surrounding dying are amplified. Unfamiliarity with personnel and medical systems magnifies uncertainty. Stress and anxiety are heightened. Everyone's fatigue deepens. Worry about the continuing physical, emotional, and financial costs compounds the situation. Dying elders' last days and weeks can be worsened significantly by the kind of emotions roiling around them. In a context of confusion and fear, it's much harder to find the emotional space to engage in the spiritual work good dying entails.

Long-proven covenants establish a stable physical, emotional, and spiritual context within which an elder can rest at ease. This ultimate sense of trust surrounds and protects a dying elder. Often for families this surrounding and holding are quite literal—touching (that most basic and intimate of the senses), embracing, resting in bed together can comfort immensely. This is the scenario of the good death—good physical and emotional care of the departing spirit.

Rail-thin, refusing to carry her oxygen equipment around in public, Marian struggled into my office on one of the few occasions she agreed to see me. Only two topics interested her now—stories of the mountains she had climbed and the Hemlock Society. She was going to die with her boots on, and by her own hand if that was what it took. That day all we accomplished was getting her advance directives on file—one important step taken. And none too soon. That very night, a new attendant panicked and called an ambulance whose crew was legally obligated when called to get the patient to the emergency room, the protests of her husband swept aside.

I received the page that Marian was en route and, knowing her clear wishes and her formal instructions, headed in to meet her and her husband at the hospital. In the emergency room, I found Bill, wringing his hands, feeling that his lifelong devotion to his wife had lapsed during the one important moment when another's fright overrode his usually implacable will. Fortunately, he had the presence of mind to bring his wife's "papers."

The anesthesiologist looked me straight in the eye. "Do you mean to say that you don't want me to insert this tube for her? Without it she is going to die right now." Bill had been kept from the room. None of this ER staff knew the kind of woman Marian was; nor had the staff heard her assure me that, when it came to dying, she "had a plan," which certainly didn't involve being kept alive on a "breathing machine." I asked that her husband join us. The hospital relented and, honoring her advance directives, left the three of us alone. Sedation calmed Marian's breathing, Bill held her hand, and she didn't last long. It was a lonely walk out for the two of us.

Making the Best of the Hospital

Back at the Station of Crisis, you came to understand just how demanding, disorienting, and difficult a hospitalization was for your sick parent—and for your family. Imagine how much more difficult it will be for an elder near death who ends up requiring, or being consigned to, hospital care. Hospitals' busy, complex environments are always difficult for elders, sick or dying. Hospitals in no way resemble a home, even to the limited extent a nursing home might. Still, we cannot predict all the circumstances of an elder's medical needs, and perhaps for symptoms that are very difficult to control (and when there is a lack of available care elsewhere), a hospital may prove the only closing option.

Many hospitals have developed palliative care services. Staffed by a dedicated team of doctors, nurses, nurse-practitioners, and others, they offer consultative services both to those with advanced illnesses and to those nearing death. These experienced and caring professionals can help guide a failing elder's transition from acute care to therapies that focus on symptom relief and comfort care (free of excessive diagnostic testing or intrusive electronic monitoring with machines). If an elder's situation becomes stable enough, a return to a more homelike setting may be best; if a situation remains unstable and transfer is difficult, a longer period of palliative care may be offered in the hospital. Usually, there will be a time limit on the use of hospital-based care, and with good reason. Hospital settings remain less peaceful, more impersonal, and more expensive than all the other care settings—home, assisted living, nursing home, or dedicated community-based hospice facilities.

Having no living relatives, eighty-seven-year-old Dr. Sarah Perkins carefully wrote up her wishes in a very precise and detailed living will and assigned a durable power of attorney for health care to Louise, a trusted social worker friend. When Sarah suffered a stroke and was taken to the hospital for evaluation on the neurology floor, I called Louise to alert her that she might be needed as a vocal advocate. When Louise arrived, she found that Sarah had suffered a massive stroke from which she was not expected to recover. Citing Sarah's express wishes, Louise got her friend discharged back to a nursing home under sensitive hospice care. For the following few weeks before her death, Sarah's friends could visit her at her bedside and offer their good-byes.

Adequate Resources

Active dying—that period of days to a few weeks at the very end—commonly involves an increasing need for care. Yet, often well-organized and available support services are scarce. An elder's needs may be in part technical—for example, more sophisticated means for providing pain relief via medication delivery pumps. Much, much more commonly, however, the need is for daily hands-on care and emotional and spiritual support. Paradoxically, in our highly medicalized system, it may be easier for a family to arrange for more technical services than for simple hands-on care. Although not everyone on your elder's advocacy team will be suited for the practical aspects of dying care, the mere presence of team members may provide the emotional and spiritual support that underlies a good death. Even in the absence of medical, nursing, or hospice support, some families with broad-enough involvement can succeed. However, the added good fortune of having medical support (perhaps an occasional home visit by a nurse or physician) can allay general anxiety and reduce uncertainty.

My older colleague had cared for this patient since the start of his practice. It was the special occasion of his own daughter's fortieth birthday that took him out of town. He asked me to cover for a few special patients over the weekend, some near death, Mrs. Fletcher among them.

Hospice hadn't yet come into favor in our small towns; such care was still family work. The call came about 9 P.M. on Saturday night, and the message was brief: "Somebody needs to see Mrs. Fletcher," was the request. Still a relatively new practitioner, I drove to the end of the road, nervous at finding so many cars around the trailer. Inside, the grandmother's bed was set up in the living room of the double-wide, with her large extended family in attendance. Mrs. Fletcher was unconscious, and long, long pauses in her breathing indicated she was merely hours from the end.

As I continued to stand by the bedside holding her hand, I confirmed for the family that the end was near. Conversation stopped. A few people nodded. I said they could call me again if they needed to and that her own doctor would be back late Sunday night. One woman thanked me for my visit, and I left.

The Slow Shutdown

Many of us caring for dying elders continue to be astonished by the slow course of dying, even when all medications (except those needed for immediate symptom relief) have been discontinued and food and fluid intake is at a minimum. For the chronically debilitated and frail, many vital systems function at a rate approximating a bare idle on a car engine. Even a very limited fuel supply of food and fluid will last for many days or, for some, many weeks. There is not a sudden end, but rather a playing out of final breaths, punctuated by extended pauses, then a return to a more stable pattern that seems unending. Even medications (such as morphine for pain relief and to ease breathing) will seldom speed or radically alter the course of passing into death.

Beyond the realm of slow shutdown is a territory occupied by more and more elders, particularly those with dementia or previous strokes who live in nursing homes. This is the protracted dying that elders supported by feeding tubes undergo. Unlike the falling-off of appetite and intake that naturally occurs near death, feeding tube solutions maintain higher nutritional reserves. In these circumstances, caregivers may have difficulty discerning when active dying actually begins. Often, there is a sense of interminable dying with no clear demarcation of change that allows a family and Circle of Concern to gather for a period of vigil and active dying care.

I had seen it often while doctoring on a remote Caribbean island: when the hospital could do nothing more, families quickly took their parent home to die. Back in the United States, the situation was a little different. After living three years in a nursing home with family visitors nearly every day, Grandmother had come to the stage of active dying. With hospice support, her family honored her wish to die at home. It turned out to be a five-day affair. All the family took time off to care for her and to be with one another. For them, it was the right, and not-too-difficult, thing to do.

Inviting Celebration

Unusual as it may sound, after long commitment and appropriate hard work, many families and groups of friends often experience a sense of celebration around an elder's expected death. A dedicated family and advocacy team create a caring and humane context for dying. An elder, ending a life with both identity and dignity intact, is at the center of everyone's attention—forgiven for what he or she did wrong or was unable to do, celebrated for a known public or lesser-known private life, and cherished in the memory of those who knew the breadth and depth of his or her being. In these intimate circumstances, family and friends both provide care and celebrate relationships, sharing stories from the past. An elder's well-supported death invites a celebration of his or her living. Expected and attended deaths connect us with a full range of human emotion. A deeply felt sense of our shared humanity helps us accept that the circle of life always closes . . . as it will one day for each of us.

The Inuit woman carefully prepares her dying mother for the sled ride out to the distant ice floe. Traditionally this last ceremony is a family affair, so she brings her two children: her son, Nanuk, age four; and her daughter, Naya, age seven. Grandmother is wrapped in warm sealskins and tenderly tied into the sled. At the end of that sad journey, she rests peacefully in the cold, white waste. After saying prayers and reluctant good-byes, the young mother and her children turn to walk home. Naya, who is old enough to understand what is happening, is very pensive. Finally, she asks, "But Mother, haven't we forgotten something? What will we use when we need a sled for you?"

—*Childhood tale, told to me by an elder friend*

Practical Tasks at the Station of Death

BEING ON THE MOUNTAINTOP

Talk About the Location of Dying and Death

When I entered practice over thirty years ago, most elders in our rural area were convinced that being admitted to the hospital was tantamount to a death sentence. They had seen the results of hospital care for the very old and quickly concluded that hospitals were way stations to death—either there or shortly after in a nursing home. To some extent, these elders weren't so very wrong. Even today, after a final passage through the hospital, nursing homes take in more and more of the dying. In 1989, 19 percent of those over age sixty-five died in a nursing home; in 1997, 24 percent; by 2020, an estimated 40 percent. Knowing this trend, I advise families to initiate discussions about a place for dying, including dying at home. These discussions may prove difficult, given our culture's attitudes toward hospitals as the location of miracles of last resort.

Recognizing our culture's reverence for technology and the wonders of scientific medicine, some have called our modern medical centers "our new cathedrals." Your family may have found consolation within these awesome halls, availing yourselves of the latest miracles for care. How painful, then, when all medical therapies for your loved one fail. Faced with your elder's transfer to the humbler surroundings of home or nursing home, you may experience a surge of both disorientation and despair. Can you look upon this new setting as a more appropriately sized chapel for the intimate, more human devotions to come? Weigh the pros and cons of location and the family work entailed in each choice. Enlist early the help of hospice or palliative care. Most families find palliative services and hospices' commitment and caring of enormous comfort in all settings—home, nursing home, and hospital.

Protracted Active Dying—The Chronic Death Standoff

The insertion of a feeding tube can honestly be described as a "minor procedure . . . done all the time." Without costly and time-consuming hands-on feeding assistance, feeding tubes help many ill patients to get a nutritional boost that promotes recovery. The clinical skills for managing feeding tubes have been easily acquired by nurses in hospitals, rehabilitation centers, and nursing homes and have speeded up the efficiency of institutional care. Today in some states, rates for feeding tube use are at 40 percent for residents of nursing homes. Other states have rates as low as 3 percent.

Although tube-feeding was initially promoted as a safer alternative to traditional hand-feeding, studies have now clearly shown that complication rates are similar for both these methods. I want to emphasize that where frail elders are concerned, we must make a distinction between what is convenient and efficient for the institution and what is humane and personal for the individual. The human touch of hands-on feeding maintains our humane connection to the person, the heart of the practice of Slow Medicine. In these devotions, families can help the staff with meals and observe any changes in a failing elder's interest and will to eat, even in those elders with dementia. Resorting to tube-feeding late in life can deny elders (and attendants) a chance to acknowledge our elders' "messages" about letting go. At this stage, it makes sense to take advantage of every possible opportunity to observe your loved one's intent in eating and living. The less we do so, the more we become distant from and oblivious to a parent's preferences for appropriate care.

Encourage Visits and Calls

Here begins your practice for life after this death. People who care about you and what you are going through will reach out, albeit tentatively, uncertain of your situation or reaction. Get comfortable with stating your preferences for talking and meeting with supportive friends. "Thanks for calling. I would love to talk with you again. Perhaps tomorrow would be better. We will know more then about how quickly she is passing." If you turn away support without expressing receptivity for later contact, you will lose opportunities not only at this station but after death occurs. Remember, what you feel emotionally this morning may be very different by this afternoon. Your reserves will wax and wane—as your parent's have done during the long journey to this moment.

Anticipatory Grieving

Living fully human lives involves experiencing both pain and joy. The longer, more intensively, and more intimately we have been involved in the care of our elders, the more we will feel their loss and see its effects. Nothing offers more depth of grieving or, paradoxically, more comfort over time than early involvement in a loved one's active care from decline through death. Although often not easy to arrange or accomplish, arriving early and staying on through the time of an elder's active dying provide family members space and time, detachment from the distractions of daily life, and adequate opportunity for reflection upon this special turning of the life cycle. Recall the extraordinary intensity of experience around the arrival of your newborn baby, from the first hours of labor through the next life-changing days, weeks, and months at home. Your life priorities assumed an essential clarity then. Now, at this final stage of a parent's life, there is again the potential for living intensely. A person's passing is not just about departing; it is about taking one's place in the long parade of generations; it is about the ceremony of passing life on to those who remain. Being present to receive this gift is paramount for honoring a life and living your own.

Language of Death

How do we find the right language when a parent is dying? In the past, the language of the deathbed was a dialect of comfort. Today, if dying takes place in the hospital, in all likelihood technical jargon will dominate because it serves the medical system so well. You cannot expect staff members at an acute-care hospital to change the way they communicate, even at a dying elder's bedside. Similarly, at home or in a nursing home, the presence of needed professional helpers will mean that some of the language of medicine will be a part of care. At times, you may find this jarring and insensitive. During the course of a person's passing, I have found there comes a gray zone where talk of "vital signs" and illness appropriately drifts toward metaphors for the long sleep of death. Quantitative medical terms ("blood pressure," "pulse rate," "oxygen saturation level"—numbers, ratios, and scales) gradually become less relevant and shift to descriptive details about an elder's overall comfort observed by the family sitting at the bedside ("relaxed," "peaceful," "sleeping"). Beyond this comes a turn to the language of the spirit, serving to remind us of the soon-to-come transition that each family will interpret according to its own spiritual and religious traditions.

Learning to Be with the Dying Person

Even for a very old person, dying can be very hard work. Failing energy and consequent fatigue make every movement and activity difficult. Breathing can become laborious. (Easing this struggle with the use of small doses of morphine can be a godsend for everyone.) Being shifted in bed to reduce pressure on fragile skin and relieve aching requires an expenditure of effort. At this station, unlike the Station of Prelude to Dying, just remaining awake and conscious enough to communicate with visitors and attendants—and respond to *their* emotions—saps the dying person physically, mentally, and emotionally.

As a family member or friend in attendance, you may have to be a gatekeeper, guiding activities and interpreting your elder's responses. Knowing "how much visiting is too much" and fending off excesses that may cause a decline in the quality of these hours may not always be easy.

Managing Anxiety

Over the past decade, much progress has been made in managing pain at the end of life. Much remains to be done, particularly as the setting for end-of-life care shifts increasingly out of the hospital. Educational efforts to accomplish this are well under way. Yet, for the very old during these last weeks of life, pain is only one of several problems needing attention: fatigue, shortness of breath, disorientation, discomforts that come with movement when the patient is attended to, dry skin and mouth, diminished bowel and bladder function. Additionally, the whole situation can be fraught with anxiety for the dying elder, for the caring family, and periodically for the overtaxed staff, including any doctors who are standing in when the patient's own doctor isn't available. Use the calming effects of touch, moderate lighting or candlelight, soft music, and gentle words. Finding ways to admit and attend to our own and others' anxieties during this period improves care immensely. Finally, if need be, tranquilizers and sedatives can be prescribed alone or in concert with pain medication to help the dying.

YOUR TEAM AT THE END

Coping with the Changing Team

A dying elder's increasing need for care in these weeks before death often means dealing with new faces and new organizations. Perhaps a hospice team (which had been mainly in support mode until now) steps in to provide more daily help. The nursing home and hospice may have worked out an arrangement whereby they coordinate care now that more bedside hours of attendance are required. Your parent's doctor and his or her covering partners are monitoring medications more closely to ensure comfort: much of this is done by telephoning and faxing, but you sense their increased involvement. Communication between groups may be so focused on formal or technical care that these new attendants may be slow to grasp who your parent was, and is.

At this closing hour, recognition of an elder's identity is more important than ever. In my own mother's experience, sharing the details of her difficult childhood enormously enriched the empathy of her minister, who attended her in the nursing home. Briefly convey information at the bedside and in hallway chats with new attendants about who your parent is and which members of the family are in attendance. The visible presence of your advocacy team helps establish a more human context for end-of-life care. Your parent is a person who matters to so many. Encourage whoever is present to engage the hospice nurse; briefly introduce yourself to the doctor dropping by.

Reach Out to Faith Communities

Some of us are active members of formal faith communities; others may have a history of lesser and stronger periods of bonding with religious groups; some of us may have neither history nor present attachment. Yet around dying there will in all likelihood be a renewed sensitivity to spiritual and religious issues, if not for you, then certainly for some members of your advocacy team and the professionals caring for your dying parent. Enormous support can be gained from religious professionals—chaplains, ministers, rabbis, and other figures—who are attached to a care facility or who have learned of a home death directly or indirectly. These caring individuals have experienced many intimate situations surrounding death. They are excellent supporters for you, your family, and the advocacy team. Ask for their involvement and draw on their support. It will help you all to share what you are feeling with those whom society has sanctioned to enter this realm of death and dying.

Initiate Contact with the Funeral Home

It was a stroke of luck for me as a young doctor to live right behind the town funeral home. My medical training with death focused on the autopsy; it certainly didn't include hearses, mortuaries, and funerals. As I got familiar with funeral homes and funeral directors, I also discovered that these men and women were a source of personal support and comfort. After-death plans sometimes get made well in advance by elders and families. At other times, they may not have been addressed at all. If you have not yet experienced a family death, you are unlikely to have met or spent time with those who will handle the body after death occurs. Early in the vigil someone will need to contact a funeral home. This can be accomplished by telephone with the help of the nursing staff. As you take needed breaks from sitting vigil (hopefully sharing rotations with other family and friends and perhaps hospice volunteers), go to the chosen funeral home and meet the people who will help your family shortly after death occurs. Spending even a few minutes to talk with them can be very reassuring and help to anchor you emotionally for those harder hours immediately after your loved one's death.

ENGAGE MEDICAL CARE

Medications in the Final Days

In the final days of life, particularly for frail elders who are shrunken by years, illness, and a falling intake of food and fluids, medications are not simply a matter of pain relief. They matter for creating a positive sense of comfort for the dying elder (and for the family at the bedside). Many deaths become "good deaths" with judicious use of regular doses of morphine and sedatives. In my experience, decisions to use such medications are always best if taken in concert with family members who can talk openly and come to agreement about both the goal of care and the degree to which they see and experience their dying parent as suffering. Decisions will also be of the highest quality if there is a constant—often hour-to-hour—review of medication use so that comfort, once achieved, is not lost by inadequate attention. Many families are surprised and pleased that so much comfort can be established with exceedingly low doses of morphine, regularly given. If your parent is not comfortable, talk to the physicians and nurses to make sure that your goals are achieved. You have every right to do so.

"Instant" Hospice

Unfortunately, many elders and their families accept the idea of hospice care only when death is imminent. And many physicians are surprisingly slow to bring it up. If your family has been fortunate in forethought, a treatment approach of palliation and a hospice program of education and active dying care have already become a consoling part of these last weeks or months of attending your parent. That said, for those elders and families for whom this hasn't already happened, there is still substantial value in requesting hospice services at the end. Because trust has such an important role in high quality of care for the dying, at this late hour there will be a need for more intensive contact and work by all to establish the bonds on which this trust is founded.

Take Away the Machines

When electrical power suddenly goes off in our homes, we become aware of how profound silence can be. No radio, no TV, no refrigerator hum. When sitting with ill loved ones in an ICU, many people find comfort in the hums and clicks of the supportive machinery of medical care. Yet many have also noted how machines can hypnotically draw attention away from the dying person. When it is clear that electronic monitoring adds nothing, and perhaps even detracts from the human focus of care, consider paring down the machinery at the bedside or in the room. When death is recognized to be near, it is not uncommon to remove even the additional oxygen coming by nasal tubes (which can dry out the nose and mouth and make them uncomfortable without offering any significant benefit). You may first experience added tranquillity, although closer to the end you will hear human sounds that will be new to you, sounds of the disordered breathing (and eventually the so-called agonal breathing) that comes as life shuts down. Quiet can make you more aware of your own feelings in these closing moments.

Share Nursing Care

Your mother's bodily needs are now being met by others. She is turned in bed regularly to protect her skin and relieve the aches that come with immobility. Her mouth is cleansed and its dryness relieved with soothing solutions. As bowel and bladder cease to function, she is monitored and cleaned as needed. Skin is washed and moistened with soothing creams and ointments. Clothing and sheets are freshly changed. All physical needs are being met. Many family attendants find their participation in some aspects of this care meaningful. For long-term home caregivers, this is simply a continuation of well-followed routines. Some of you may want a role that expresses your love and relieves the work of others. Established through the intimacy of touch, the memory of your hands-on care will long remain with you. After death, attendants customarily care for the body of the deceased, doing a final bathing or cleansing and perhaps redressing and rearranging the body to a position that looks more comfortable. Traditionally, of course, families have always washed and dressed the bodies of their dead. I have known individuals who found much meaning and comfort in returning to this age-old tradition. The caregiving staff should be open to this sort of participation, or persuaded to be receptive.

. . .

DYING AND DEATH precipitate our most intense emotional and psychological responses. Witness any news photo of a grieving parent, son, or daughter at the site of an accidental death. With an elder's slower dying and expected death, there may not be the same spontaneous intensity and outpouring of feeling, but the same profound emotional, mental, and spiritual forces are there, lying in wait. Preparation for loss may alter how you grieve, but these latent human forces will need to be reckoned with.

You may be caught off guard in institutions such as hospitals and nursing homes, where death is a frequent and familiar occurrence. You may find yourself offended by the staff's casual use of the term "expected death," conveying to you the message that the experience should be easier. It may be "routine" for the staff members, who find ways to cope and protect themselves from the regular and repeated feelings of loss that they experience, but it will not, even after so many months and years of tending, be so for you.

Watch out for behaving as you imagine others see fit. Relief, peace, sadness, anger may suddenly flare—people's responses are unpredictable. Even if we as family, doctors, nurses, and other caregivers have done this work well and successfully, seldom will we feel the same sense of triumph that comes with other types of work well done. Even if feelings are not being openly expressed, know that others, at some level, are sharing your loss.

Grieving/Legacy

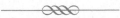

"We did the right things . . ."
—BROTHER

In a moment our elder's "presence" turns to "past," and the story shifts to us—the surviving family. Stories of loss come back so predictably each time grief enters our lives. My sister and I bring memories deeply anchored in our childhoods, grieving for an absent and unknown father. After that they diverge. Most of mine have accumulated in my life as a doctor; hers have been more personal. As a medical student early in training, I was the member of our ward team assigned the task of turning off the ventilator of an old Lithuanian man who was terminally unconscious with heart failure. Although I had cared for him from the moment of his arrival in the emergency room four days before, I felt strangely detached as he took his last few breaths without the support of the machine.

A year later, as an intern, I wept alone and uncontrollably in the stairwell after the ventilator was discontinued for my ten-year-old patient who had accidentally hanged himself. All the deaths experienced during my first years of becoming a doctor were grieved with those wrenching tears—as were the deaths of my grandfather and father. My losses accumulate and flow together.

Seldom shorter than months and often lasting for years or the rest of a lifetime, this final station requires both space and time to be accomplished. After an early period of keen emotional and physical intensity, much of our grieving around a loved one's death takes place over a much longer period of time.

> *From "Shapes"*
> In the longer view it doesn't matter.
> However, it's that having lived, it matters,
> so that every death breaks you apart.
> You find yourself weeping at the door
> of your own kitchen, overwhelmed
> at loss. And you find yourself weeping
> as you pass the homeless person
> head in hands resigned on a cement
> step, the wire basket on wheels right there.
>
> —RUTH STONE

Being with the Body

For most family members and friends, grieving began a long time before a loved one's death. Once our parents enter late life, we become increasingly aware of their changed selves and growing losses. Now we face something different—their ongoing absence.

As an elder breathes his or her last breaths, the transition to absence of life in the body is relatively sudden. No movement. No sound. A subtle change in skin color. Many in attendance experience this time as having a dimension beyond the minutes surrounding the final breath.

In the silence that follows, the presence of your loved one can linger for some time before there is a feeling of a further departure. After death has come, there is no reason for any rush to move the deceased. If you have been able to create a quiet context for dying, it can serve very well as the place for saying a final good-bye and continuing the process of grieving. In my experience, many family members and friends who were near at the time of death want to spend some private moments—perhaps together, but more often alone—with the body of their loved one. After such intense and committed involvement, many nonfamily caregivers also wish to pay their respects or say good-bye in a moment of quietness. Yet, being with the body may not serve all well; it is a highly personal decision, often not made until the actual moment of choosing. Regardless of choice, in these quiet moments, we begin to experience an altered sense of time and orientation that will govern our lives for at least the near future.

Family members, friends, and caregivers should feel free to linger. Hours may be allowed to pass before any real need to move the body arises, and even then it is more to support the process of moving on. If you feel rushed in any way, you should be aware that this has nothing to do with any requirement of caring for the deceased, but more to do with logistics—for instance, changing of shifts in a nursing home, needing to free a bed in the hospital. Be aware that different family members have different emotional needs: prolonging this time of sitting with the body may help some and may be distressing to others.

As widely noted for most of us, the immediate period after death carries some sense of disbelief and unreality. Because disbelief prevails, early tears may be softer than the hard waves of acute physical grief that may wash over us periodically for months and months. For now, a swirl of activity takes over—notifying distant relatives and friends, greeting intimates, connecting with the funeral home, preparing for the funeral or memorial service. For family members at a distance, the journey "home" begins. We are swept through the blur of the next several days before finding ourselves alone after the completed formalities of our cultural practices surrounding death.

Beginning the Longer Journey: a Return to Slow Medicine's Foundation

LIFE CYCLES AND INDIVIDUALS

What can be more personal than the way each of us grieves? If your parent has lived a long life, you have probably watched a downhill spiral that in some ways softens grief. For my sister and me, Mother was, like those old trees that finally fall, beyond her full maturity. Her life had indeed been full. But, inevitably, her interest in the present and connections to the future faded away. Difficult as it was not to want just a little more of her before having to shift to the gifts of memory, we finally were able to let go of our hope for any small potential that might remain in her tired body. Along with our grief, we felt relief and gratitude that she had been delivered at last from her shrunken life, and the ever-present threats of more debilitation and suffering.

With sudden deaths, even for elders, we are often left with the feeling that there was so much more life to be lived "if only this hadn't happened." When a person's death is premature, we intensely grieve their lost human potential. The haunting sorrow of unmet expectations remains—"She never saw her grandson graduate from college"; "She never knew that her granddaughter was pregnant." This kind of loss, experienced as a kind of violence, can lead to a different kind of grieving that puts one at a higher risk for depression. How different from the grieving and celebration of potential all expended.

"We still have Mother" was the comforting refrain my sister and I would tell ourselves over Mother's long lifetime. But once we lost our second parent, we came to understand emotionally that the generational baton had passed to us. This final familial loss forces adult children to confront their own mortality on a completely different level.

ACKNOWLEDGING COVENANTAL RELATIONSHIPS

As you look back, you will undoubtedly become more appreciative of those who came and stayed and helped. Perhaps you will want to thank a parent's physician or acknowledge the "surrogate" covenantal roles faithfully played by others. Your sister or sister-in-law, the caregivers who tended your parent for months or years—all may have enacted a role of caring and commitment that transcended simple family bonds or expectations. And remember the group of care providers who sustained the supportive intimacy nurturing your parent when the immediate family could not be present. There is often a need to bring to a formal end this "temporary family." The personal work of caregiving often breaks hearts and makes losses deeply felt. The courtesy of acknowledging one another's contributions as we move on in our lives is vital to securing the maturation gained from our experience.

As you say your thanks; acknowledge condolences and the service of others; complete final paperwork; clean out a house, apartment, or room; disburse possessions; and settle an estate, you will begin to recognize what you will take with you emotionally. Your covenant involves carrying forward the essence of an elder's life and identity into the future. You are pivotal in determining what will be passed on. Some of this giving may have happened gradually over years or even decades as elders have transferred cherished physical possessions to family members. Now you may use the deeper insights into character that you have gained over these final years of reconnecting, reevaluating, forgiving, and caring to hold true to your covenant with your deceased loved one. Remember and eulogize all that was admirable—his or her stoicism, gentle kindness, friendly acceptance of others, lack of vanity, and love of dancing. Perhaps your covenant takes the larger form of carrying out broader wishes for the family or defending the values your parent stood for that you also share. Devoting ourselves to this work enriches the course of our lives. At the same time, fulfilling this work helps us forge the personal covenants we will need to support the process of our own aging and eventual death.

INTERDEPENDENCY

"Currents of remembrance" now dominate our days. Memories and "conversations" come out of nowhere. Responses are triggered by many things—familiar scenes, possessions left in a drawer, the smells of clothing as we empty closets, a song we hear on the radio, photographs, and simple passing thoughts. Brief but vivid hallucinations may occur as we catch a glimpse of Mother, or Dad tells us that he "feels that she is still around the house." Spouses report turning over in bed and sensing that a longtime partner shifted in response.

At the same time that these ghostly connections so permeate our awareness, we move through the larger world with an "unworn badge." So many of our culture's formal practices of grieving have disappeared. We no longer don the dark dress of grieving; nor do we stay in seclusion or hold extended wakes. We often must return to distant homes and are not available for the traditional round of visits from local friends and family members. Indeed, after our time away, we are expected to return quickly to our own lives—resuming regular routines with the family, at work, and with friends. "It was good you could be there at the end," say consoling colleagues, but for you it is by no means over. Still, in a society so tightly scheduled, we feel pressed to conform to social and work expectations. After all, many others seem to have quickly gotten over a death. Be prepared for a rapid closing of the waters of feeling outside the immediate family.

For our grieving to proceed and legacies to be established, time and space are still required. Do we prefer to create our own personal rituals—with readings, prayers, and candles—or do we gravitate to our own religious communities or simply to our closest friends for comfort? In the Caribbean, every holiday and family celebration is graced by a shrine of "parent's plate," food and drink surrounded by photographs and candles in a quiet back bedroom—ongoing remembrance of the dead.

Will those who so stoically carried the burden of months or years of caring and gradual losses find less acceptance from others when strong physical surges of grief unexpectedly recur? Do men and women grieve differently, making this period even more lonely and emotionally difficult or discordant? Do we label ourselves "weak" or "out of control" because of our continuing emotional interdependency? Just as you gathered an advocacy team for your parent, you may feel a need for your own support team. You may now commune with a heightened understanding of your friends' losses. All the while you are modeling modes of empathy—strength for your own children and their eventual carrying of someone else up the mountain.

COMMUNICATION

If you have done your job well, you have devoted a great deal of time to building communication skills, establishing networks of caring, and learning how to talk with other family members and with the array of outsiders required for your loved one's care. Using both verbal and nonverbal communication, you made sure that necessary information was carefully passed back and forth to benefit your parent.

Now that the immediate activities required by a death are behind you, you may find yourself in a space of resounding quiet. Increasingly, communication becomes internal—monologues with yourself or perhaps bits of unfinished conversations with your parent. Accept the importance of these "internal talks," until you learn to condense and share some of what is going on inside you.

Mourners also communicate through their activities. We model grief and celebration for our children and grandchildren and those less experienced with loss than we have become. We tell the important stories of our legacy and perhaps spend time tidying up, ascribing names and dates to books of photos and other mementos communicating a life to succeeding generations. Perhaps we make a communal donation to our parent's favorite charity or create an heirloom recipe book or undertake for posterity a family tree-planting ceremony.

REACH OUT TO OTHERS

The kindness of others supports our grieving, patiently allowing us time and space to articulate and incorporate our loss and then to gradually become reintegrated into life around us. Despite the daily emotional ups and downs we exhibit following a death, our friends usually risk treading into this uncertain territory to reach out to us. Because we have turned inward to do our emotional work, it may be easy to neglect or overlook these small extensions of kindness, thereby inhibiting further overtures to share and support. Although often difficult during this time of active grieving, receptivity and showing up in response to invitations are important for our own health. It becomes all too easy to slide out of friends' lives. This can be particularly dangerous for your widowed mother or father.

Also looming large during this period of grieving is the gradual and natural reemergence of old conflicts and difficult memories as the eulogizing ends. Many of us are part of wounded families, some of us with isolated personal wounds going back decades, perhaps to childhood. We may still cry inwardly, despite all the work we have done to heal and forgive during our period of caring for our parents. We are left with a mixture of good and not-so-good gifts as a part of our legacy, and our personal journey achieves a recognition that only forgiveness and kindness can bring about the final healing that comes with the passing of our loved one's life.

"Peace My Heart"

Peace, my heart, let the time for the parting be sweet.

Let it not be a death but completeness.

Let love melt into memory and pain into songs.

Let the flight through the sky end in the folding of the wings over
the nest.

Let the last touch of your hand be gentle like the flower of the
night.

Stand still, O Beautiful End, for a moment, and say your last words
in silence.

I bow to you and hold up my lamp to light you on your way.

—RABINDRANATH TAGORE

Over all the long and difficult months and years of sharing our parent's journey to the mountaintop, we have changed and matured in the depths of our understanding. The view from that passing height of human experience reorders priorities. Our deep identification with the frailty and the needs of a dying loved one awakens in us a new capacity for compassion. Our daily practice of caring has deepened our humanity. Bringing these changes forward into our own lives enriches our relationships and seeds the covenantal ground from which our own future well-being will grow. A good death for our parent means a better life for us.

Epilogue

—June 18, 2007

Late-life journeys are surely unpredictable . . . to the very end. My mother, Bertha McCullough, died at age ninety-two at Omega House, a residential hospice in Houghton, Michigan, on April 24, 2007. Her faithful physicians, very ably supplemented by the staff at the home and by the Keweenaw Home Health and Hospice team, cared for her to the end. Her minister and her church extended enormous support to her and to us, her family. She died twenty miles from where she was born and within five miles of every residence she ever occupied.

The unexpected twist at the end, which was a gift and totally outside our planning, was the suggestion by the hospice team that she be transferred from the nursing home where she had lived for eighteen months after giving up her senior apartment. The routines and support by the nursing home staff, who had served her so commendably over that too-long (in my mother's eyes) stay, became a daily, disorienting burden for her—too often awakened out of sleep, too many offers of food, too much expected of her in her exhaustion. She finally cried out, "Why is dying so hard to do?"

Then she was blessed with the gift of a room at Omega House, a recently built community-run residential hospice. Although unsure if she had the strength to make the short transfer from the nursing home (and at times disoriented as to what it meant to move), she survived the change. All medications, except a small dose of minor pain reliever directed toward her comfort, were stopped. After sleeping nearly twenty-four hours immediately after arrival and leaving us in fear that she might never awaken again, she opened her eyes and asked for a cup of coffee and an egg "over easy." Over the next five weeks Bertha established her own rhythm of twenty-two hours of sleep each day and a couple of hours of time awake during which she ate a small meal when and if she wanted it. We carefully followed her small clues to meet her needs and desires. Each day she awoke in beautiful new and peaceful homelike surroundings. A low window allowed her to see the nearby woods from her bed; two recliners gave us comfortable resting places beside her bed. Her mental clarity returned. She spoke to us of her dreams, her dying, and her funeral. She regained her humor and appreciated her attendants. Our family experienced a return of "quality time" together.

Why did this final leg of the journey work so well for Bertha and for us? Years of "showing up," traveling long distances for what were often only short visits, had allowed us to forge relationships with caregivers who sustained her when we were not there. Bertha's identity remained intact, and she held on to her dignity, despite becoming so very dependent on others to get through the day. Over many, many months and years, trust was forged that eventually allowed her and us, other attendants, professionals, and friends to feel that we all shared her caretaking and that each of us would predictably and reliably do his or her part. As we became sure of one another's commitment, our growing confidence was communicated among us, more through actions than through words. This trust also allowed for the individual compromises that are often necessary during such prolonged journeys. Upholding a track record of making good day-to-day decisions, we practiced doing the right small things over and over through years of mounting difficulty.

Slow Medicine is just this caring process of slowing down, being patient, coordinating care, and remaining faithful to the end. Families necessarily bear the greatest responsibility in surmounting difficulties to create this bond of trust and security for their loved ones. Over and over, families must identify and ask for what they and their parents need, seeking links to caring professionals who also want to do the right thing, but are often constrained by organizational, institutional, and cultural health care practices that are not fully serving our elders and us . . . yet.

Now, as waves of sadness and loss wash over us from day to day since her death, our pain is tempered by our satisfaction and pride in having done right by our mother through to the end of her long life. Our gratitude for the loving care she so selflessly gave to us has been enriched and deepened by our memories of the grace and patience with which she taught us how to die a good death. May we do half so well when our own journeys to the mountaintop begin.

Slow Medicine Websites

These key websites will lead you to a wealth of others through their links.

www.aafp.org: American Academy of Family Physicians—use "patients" tab and then go to "seniors" section for medical information.

www.aahsa.org: American Association of Homes and Services for the Aging—use "Aging Services: The Facts" and "Consumer Information" for housing and services information.

www.aarp.org: The American Association of Retired Persons—broad range of health and aging resources and links.

www.alzheimers.org: National Institute on Aging website—addresses Alzheimer's comprehensively.

www.americangeriatrics.org: The American Geriatric Society—use "patient education" and "health links."

www.caregiver.org: Family Caregiver Alliance and National Center on Caregiving—useful information on caregiving issues.

www.caringinfo.org: National Hospice and Palliative Care Organization website—family and patient education and resources.

www.cms.hhs.gov: Official Medicare website—start with the more readable *Medicare and You Handbook*.

www.healthinaging.org: American Geriatric Society Foundation for Health in Aging website—see "Eldercare at Home" guide.

www.nfcacares.org: National Family Caregiver Association—excellent support resource.

www.npaonline.org: National PACE Association—to locate PACE programs.

Slow Medicine Reading

Here are a few recommended books to start you out on a journey of reading about aging.

Dying Well: The Prospect for Growth at the End of Life (Putnam/Riverhead, 1997) by Ira Byock, M.D. Stories from the end of life.

Ethical Wills: Putting Your Values on Paper (Perseus, 2002), by Barry Baines, M.D. Helpful guide to engaging this work of reflection.

Healthy Aging: A Lifelong Guide to Your Physical and Spiritual Well-Being (HarperCollins, 2006), by Andrew Wiel, M.D. A "pre-elder guide" to Slow Medicine.

Island: The Collected Stories (Random House, 2000), by Alistair MacLeod. Great range of intergenerational family stories, including the ultimate "holding-out" story.

Now and Then: Poems 1976–1978 (Random House, 1978), by Robert Penn Warren. Pulitzer Prize–winning volume of poems from late life.

The Oxford Book on Aging: Reflections on the Journey of Life (Oxford University Press, 1994), Thomas Cole, editor. A broad look at the long literature of aging.

The 36-Hour Day: A Family Guide to Caring for Persons with Alzheimer's Disease, Related Dementing Illnesses, and Memory Loss in Later Life (Johns Hopkins University Press, 1991), by Nancy Mace and Peter Rabins, M.D. Still the classic, years later.

The Year of Magical Thinking (Knopf, 2005), by Joan Didion. An account of being deeply inside grief.

Slow Medicine Cinema

An easy entry into the world of elders is through these gentle, deeply feeling, and often funny portrayals of aging. Here are some of my favorites.

Umberto D. (1952, Dir. Vittorio De Sica). Vittorio De Sica directs a poignant story of an elderly widower and his dog.

Smultronstället (Wild Strawberries). (1957, Dir. Ingmar Bergman). Bergman classic on an aging physician reconciling a life.

On Golden Pond (1981, Dir. Mark Rydell). American intergenerational classic featuring Katharine Hepburn, a crusty Henry Fonda, and, playing his rebellious daughter, Jane Fonda.

The Trip to Bountiful (1985, Dir. Peter Masterson). Geraldine Page in an Academy Award–winning role of a widow "returning home" in search of happier memories.

Foxfire (1987, Dir. Jud Taylor). The acclaimed husband-and-wife acting team of Hume Cronyn and Jessica Tandy, in a story of a widow "holding out" in her family home.

The Whales of August (1987, Dir. Lindsay Anderson). Aging Bette Davis and Lillian Gish summering on the New England coast in a timeless culture.

Stanno Tutti Bene (Everybody's Fine) (1990, Dir. Giuseppe Tornatore). Marcello Mastroianni plays a recent widower reconnecting with his children, all of whom have secrets they want to keep.

Strangers in Good Company (1990, Dir. Cynthia Scott). A stranded busload of elders sharing stories and lives during a crisis in the wilderness.

Wrestling Ernest Hemingway (1993, Dir. Randa Haines). Old men evolving. A dapper dentist played by Robert Duvall befriends Richard Harris's roaring sailor, with Sandra Bullock in a charming supporting role.

To Dance with the White Dog (1993, Dir. Glenn Jordan). Again, Hume Cronyn and Jessica Tandy explore the world of grief.

Buena Vista Social Club (1999, Dir. Wim Wenders). Music, aging, and pure joy. Ry Cooder's loving tribute to joyous and still-playing Cuban musical legends.

The Straight Story (1999, Dir. David Lynch). An unusually "straight" story directed by David Lynch. With no driver's license and the need to mend a family relationship, Richard Farnsworth takes a lawn mower journey across the Midwest.

Innocence (2000, Dir. Paul Cox). Love is ageless, so they say, and this moving love story for elders explores the consequences.

Iris (2001, Dir. Richard Eyre). Judi Dench and Jim Broadbent in an exploration of a rich life together ending in Iris Murdoch's descent into Alzheimer's disease.

About Schmidt (2002, Dir. Alexander Payne). A grieving widower, played by Jack Nicholson, mourns his losses and starts again in surprising ways. A searching look at American male aging.

Secondhand Lions (2003, Dir. Tim McCanlies). Sometimes the stories your eccentric old "uncles" tell are true. Robert Duvall and Michael Caine mentor a boy to manhood.

Mrs. Palfrey at the Claremont (2005, Dir. Dan Ireland). Joan Plowright gives a sparkling performance in this comedy about a widow's new friendship in a "senior" hotel.

Aurora Borealis (2005, Dir. James C. E. Burke). Donald Sutherland in an exceptional performance as an elder coping with illness.

Bibliography

Abramson, J. *Overdosed America: The Broken Promise of American Medicine*. New York: HarperCollins, 2004.

Adams, J., and L. Gerson. "A New Model for Emergency Care of Geriatric Patients." *Academic Emergency Medicine* 10 (2003): 271–274.

Ahmed, A., and R. Sims. "Demographic Characteristics of U.S. Nursing Homes and Their Residents: Highlights of the National Nursing Home Survey, 1995." *Annals of Long-Term Care* 8 (2000): 62–67.

American Geriatrics Society and Association of Directors of Geriatric Academic Programs. *Geriatric Medicine: A Clinical Imperative for an Aging Population*. New York: American Geriatrics Society, 2004.

American Geriatrics Society Health Care Systems Committee. "Assisted Living Facilities: American Geriatrics Society Position Paper." *Journal of the American Geriatrics Society* 53:3 (2005): 536–537.

Angelelli, J. "Promising Models for Transforming Long-Term Care." *The Gerontologist* 46 (2006): 428–430.

Back, A., and R. Arnold. "Dealing with Conflict in Caring for the Seriously Ill: 'It Was Just Out of the Question,' " *Journal of the American Medical Association* 293 (2005): 1374–1381.

Baines, B. *Ethical Wills: Putting Your Values on Paper*. New York: Perseus, 2002.

Beers, M. "Explicit Criteria for Determining Potentially Inappropriate Medication Use by the Elderly: An Update." *Archives of Internal Medicine* 48 (1997): 1289–1296.

Belluck, P. "As Minds Age, What's Next? Brain Calisthenics Surge." *New York Times,* Dec. 27, 2006.

Benefield, L. E. "Long-Distance Family Caregiving for Frail Elders." *Gerontological Society of America Annual Meeting 2005 Paper Abstracts,* 89.

Bergmann, M., et al. "Delerium Persistence in Patients Admitted to Post-Acute Skilled Nursing Facilities." *American Geriatrics Society Annual Meeting 2003 Paper Abstracts,* S29.

Boling, P. "Using Home Care to Improve Outcomes and Lower Costs." *Clinical Geriatrics* 12 (2004): 30–35.

Boockvar, K., and D. Meier. "Palliative Care for Frail Older Adults: 'There Are Things I Can't Do Anymore That I Wish I Could . . .' " *Journal of the American Medical Association* 29 (2006): 2245–2253.

Boult, C., and J. Pacala. "Integrating Healthcare for Older Populations." *American Journal of Managed Care* 5 (1999): 45–52.

Boyd, C., et al. "Clinical Practice Guidelines and Quality of Care for Older Patients with Multiple Comorbid Diseases: Implications of Pay for Performance." *Journal of the American Medical Association* 294 (2005): 716–724.

Brach, J., et al. "The Association Between Physical Function and Lifestyle Activity and Exercise in the Health, Aging, and Body Composition Study." *Journal of the American Geriatrics Society* 52 (2004): 502–509.

Branch, Laurence G., ed. "Integration of Care in a Changing Environment." Special issue, *Generations* 23:2 (1999).

Brody, J. "Medical Due Diligence: A Living Will Should Spell Out Specifics." *New York Times,* Nov. 28, 2006.

Brummel-Smith, K. "A Gastrostomy in Every Stomach?" *Journal of the American Board of Family Practice* 11 (1998): 242–243.

Buettner, Dan. "The Secrets of Living Longer." *National Geographic Magazine,* Nov. 2005.

Burton, A., et al. "Bereavement After Caregiving or Unexpected Death: Effects on Elderly Spouses." *Gerontological Society of America Annual Meeting 2005 Paper Abstracts,* 207.

Butcher, H., and M. McGoigal-Kenney. "Living in the Doldrums: Experiencing Dispiritedness in Later Life." *Gerontological Society of America Annual Meeting 2005 Paper Abstracts,* 358.

Carpenter, G. I. "Aging in the United Kingdom and Europe—A Snapshot of the Future?" *Journal of the American Geriatrics Society* 53 (2005): S309–S313.

Cassel, C. *Medicare Matters: What Geriatric Medicine Can Teach American Health Care.* Berkeley: University of California Press, 2005.

Center for the Evaluative Clinical Sciences. *The Dartmouth Atlas of Health Care 2005.* Chicago: American Hospital Publishing Company, 2006.

Cesari, M., et al. "Prevalence and Risk Factors for Falls in an Older Community-Dwelling Population." *Journals of Gerontology Series A: Biological Sciences and Medical Sciences* 57 (2002): 722–726.

Charette, S. "The Next Step: Palliative Care for Advanced Heart Failure." *Journal of the American Medical Directors Association* 6 (2005): 63–64.

Chaudhry, S., et al. "Systolic Hypertension in Older Persons." *Journal of the American Medical Association* 292 (2004): 1074–1080.

Chodosh, J., et al. "Cognitive Decline in High-Functioning Older Persons Is Associated with an Increased Risk of Hospitalization." *Journal of the American Geriatrics Society* 52 (2004): 1456–1462.

Chuang, Tzu. "Dialogues." In *The Oxford Book of Aging,* ed. Thomas R. Cole and Mary G. Winkler, 80–81. New York: Oxford University Press, 1994.

Clarfield, A. "Paying with Interest for a High Interest in Screening." *Journal of the American Geriatrics Society* 54 (2006): 1465–1466.

Cora, V. "Helping Family Caregivers of Older Adults with Dementia." *ElderCare* 6 (2006): 1–4.

Corbet, B. "Embedded: Nursing Home Undercover." *AARP Magazine,* Jan.–Feb. 2007, 82–100.

Corrigan, B. "Therese Schroeder-Shaker—Music Thanatology and Spiritual Care for the Dying." *Alternative Therapies* 7 (2001): 69–77.

Crecelius, C., and S. Levenson. "Cholinesterase Inhibitors: Appropriate Uses in Long-Term Care." *Caring for the Ages* 5 (2004): 28–29.

Creditor, M. "Hazards of Hospitalization of the Elderly." *Annals of Internal Medicine* 118 (1993): 219–223.

Davis, J., et al. "Improving Transition and Communication Between Acute Care and Long-Term Care: A System for Better Continuity of Care." *Annals of Long-Term Care* 13 (2005): 25–32.

DeJonge, E., et al. "How Does a Medical House Call Program Affect Health Care Utilization?" *American Geriatric Society Annual Meeting 2003 Paper Abstracts,* S225.

Division of Geriatric Medicine, Saint Louis University School of Medicine. "End-of-Life Care: Moving Towards the Ideal." *Aging Successfully* 16:1 (2006): 12–13.

———. "Taking Medications: Benefits and Risks." *Aging Successfully* 13:3 (2003): 2.

Dolara, A. "Invito ad una 'slow medicine.'" *Italian Heart Journal* 30 (2003): 100–101.

Dosa, D. "Should I Hospitalize My Resident with Nursing Home–Acquired Pneumonia." *Journal of the American Medical Directors Association* 6 (2005): 327–333.

Dossey, L. "Forgetting." *Alternative Therapies* 8 (2002): 12–16, 103–107.

Doukas, D., and J. Hardwig. "Using the Family Covenant in Planning End-of-Life Care: Obligations and Promises of Patients, Families, and Physicians." *Journal of the American Geriatrics Society* 51 (2003): 1155–1158.

Doust, J., and C. Del Mar. "Why Do Doctors Use Treatments That Do Not Work? For Many Reasons—Including Their Inability to Stand Idle and Do Nothing." *British Medical Journal–USA* 4 (2004): 209–210.

Drane, J. *Becoming a Good Doctor: The Place of Virtue and Character in Medical Ethics.* Lanham, MD: Sheed and Ward, 1988.

Drinka, P., and C. Crnich. "Pneumonia in the Nursing Home." *Journal of the American Medical Directors Association* 6 (2005): 342–350.

Eastman, P. "Forecast: More Long-Term Care Options for Low-Income Americans." *Caring for the Ages* 4 (July 2003): 1.

Flaherty, J., et al. "The Development of Outpatient Clinical Guidepaths." *Journal of the American Geriatrics Society* 50 (2002): 1886–1901.

Franco, O., et al. "The Polymeal: A More Natural, Safer, and Probably Tastier (Than the Polypill) Strategy to Reduce Cardiovascular Disease by More Than 75%." *British Medical Journal–USA* 5 (2005): 71–74.

Freedman, V., et al. "Recent Trends in Disability and Functioning Among Older Adults in the United States." *Journal of the American Medical Association* 288 (2002): 3137–3146.

Freund, B., and F. Segal-Gidan. "The Older Adult Driver: Issues and Concerns for the Geriatric Physician." *Annals of Long-Term Care* 9 (2003): 37–39.

Fries, J. "Reducing Disability in Older Age." *Journal of the American Medical Association* 288 (2002): 3164–3166.

Galanos, A., and K. Elbert-Avila. "Palliative Care in Long-Term Care: Communicating with Families." *Annals of Long-Term Care* 12 (2004): 26–32.

Gessert, C., et al. "Dying of Old Age: An Examination of Death Certificates of Minnesota Centenarians." *Journal of the American Geriatrics Society* 50 (2002): 1561–1565.

Gill, T., et al. "Hospitalization, Restricted Activity, and the Development of Disability Among Older Persons." *Journal of the American Medical Association* 292 (2004): 2115–2124.

Goldstein, N., and S. Morrison. "The Intersection Between Geriatrics and Palliative Care: A Call for a New Research Agenda." *Journal of the American Geriatrics Society* 53 (2005): 1593–1598.

Gordon, M. "CPR in Long-Term Care: Mythical Benefits or Necessary Ritual?" *Annals of Long-Term Care* 11 (2003): 41–49.

Greene, K. "Aging Well: To Get a Parent to the Doctor, Watch Your Bedside Manner." *Wall Street Journal,* Dec. 9, 2003.

____. "Is There a Doctor in the House: It's Becoming Tougher to Find—and Keep—the Medical Providers You Need in Later Life, Particularly in Retirement Hot Spots." *Wall Street Journal,* Aug. 21, 2006.

Greene, M., et al. "Concordance Between Physicians and Their Older and Younger Patients in the Primary Care Medical Encounter." *The Gerontologist* 29 (1989): 808–813.

Greene, R. "And Then It Happens to You: When Professional and Personal Roles Intersect." *Gerontological Society of America Annual Meeting 2005 Paper Abstracts,* 303–304.

Gross, J. "As Parents Age, Baby Boomers and Business Struggle to Cope." *New York Times,* Mar. 25, 2006.

_____. "Geriatrics Lags in the Age of High-Tech Medicine." *New York Times,* Oct. 18, 2006.

Grumbach, K. "Chronic Illness, Comorbidities, and the Need for Medical Generalism." *Annals of Family Medicine* 1:1 (2003): 4–7.

Halpern, S., and J. Hansen-Flaschen. "Terminal Withdrawal of Life-Sustaining Supplemental Oxygen." *Journal of the American Medical Association* 296 (2006): 1397–1400.

Hampton, T. "Urinary Catheter Use Often 'Inappropriate' in Hospitalized Elderly Patients." *Journal of the American Medical Association* 295 (2006): 2838.

Hansen, L., and M. Ersek. "Meeting Palliative Care Needs in Post-Acute Care Settings: 'To Help Them Live Until They Die.' " *Journal of the American Medical Association* 295 (2006): 681–686.

Hardy, S., and T. Gill. "Recovery from Disability Among Community-Dwelling Older Persons." *Journal of the American Medical Association* 291 (2004): 1596–1602.

Harris, R. "Screening for Glaucoma: Waiting Until Our Vision Clears." *British Medical Journal–USA* 5 (2005): 381–382.

Herring, H. "Boomers Hit 60, Supporting Both Young and Old." *New York Times,* Jan. 8, 2006.

Hickman, S., et al. "Use of the Physician Orders for Life-Sustaining Treatment Program in Oregon Nursing Facilities: Beyond Resuscitation Status." *Journal of the American Geriatrics Society* 52 (2004): 1424–1429.

Hirschman, K., et al. "Hospice in Long-Term Care." *Annals of Long-Term Care* 13:10 (2005): 25–29.

Hoffman, J. "The Last Word on the Last Breath." *New York Times,* Oct. 10, 2006.

Honore, C. *In Praise of Slowness: How a Worldwide Movement Is Challenging the Cult of Speed.* New York: HarperCollins, 2004.

Hussey, J. "Creating Lasting Legacies Through Life Story Writing." *Journal on Active Aging* 5 (2006): 58–64.

Inouye, S., et al. "The Hospital Elder Life Program: A Model of Care to Prevent Cognitive and Functional Decline in Older Hospitalized Patients." *Journal of the American Geriatrics Society* 48 (2000): 1697–1706.

Intrator, O., et al. "Nursing Home Characteristics and Potentially Preventable Hospitalization of Long-Stay Residents." *Journal of the American Geriatrics Society* 52 (2004): 1730–1736.

Johansson, J., et al. "Natural History of Early, Localized Prostate Cancer." *Journal of the American Medical Association* 291 (2004): 2713–2719.

Jones, J. "Assessments for Older Adults." *IDEA Health and Fitness Source,* Jan. 2000, 75–81.

Journal of the American Medical Association. "Executive Summary of the Third Report of the National Cholesterol Education Program Expert Panel on Detection, Evaluation, and Treatment of High Blood Cholesterol in Adults." *Journal of the American Medical Association* 285 (2001): 2486–2497.

Kaduszkiewicz, H., et al. "Cholinesterase Inhibitors for Patients with Alzheimer's Disease: Systematic Review of Randomized Clinical Trials." *British Medical Journal–USA* 5 (2005): 459–462.

Kane, R. "Losing Neverland: Creating a Better World to Age In." *Journal of the American Medical Directors Association* 6 (2005): 353–356.

Kane, R., and J. West. *It Shouldn't Have to Be This Way.* Nashville, TN: Vanderbilt University Press, 2005.

Kapo, J., and D. Casarett. "Prognosis in Chronic Diseases." *Annals of Long-Term Care* 14:2 (2006): 18–23.

Kapp, M. "Medical Mistakes and Older Patients: Admitting Errors and Improving Care." *Journal of the American Geriatrics Society* 49 (2001): 1361–1365.

Karch, B., et al. "Social Factors in Health Promotion." *Health Promotion: Global Perspectives,* 3 (2000): 1–8.

Katz, P., and J. Karuza. "Physician Practice in Nursing Homes." *Journal of the American Medical Directors Association* 7 (2006): 393–398.

Kübler-Ross, E. *On Death and Dying.* New York: Macmillan, 1969.

Kumar, P. "Study Highlights the Most Effective Treatments of NPS (Neuropsychiatric Symptoms) of Dementia: Teaching Caregivers How to Interact with Patients Tops the List of Psychological Therapies." *Caring for the Ages* 7 (2006): 12.

Lamont, E., and N. Christakis. "Complexities in Prognosis in Advanced Cancer: 'To Help Them Live Their Lives the Way They Want To.' " *Journal of the American Medical Association* 290 (2003): 98–104.

LaRosa, J., et al. "Unanswered Questions: The Use of Statins in Older People to Prevent Cardiovascular Event—Effects of Statins on Risk of Coronary Disease: A Meta-Analysis of Randomized Controlled Trials." *Journal of the American Geriatrics Society* 50 (2002): 391–393.

Leutz, W., M. Greenlick, and L. Nonnenkamp. *Linking Medical Care and Community Services: Practical Models for Bridging the Gap.* New York: Springer, 2003.

Levenson, S., and F. Feinsod. "Determining Decision-Making Capacity and Selecting a Primary Decision-Maker." *Annals of Long-Term Care* 6 (1998): 370–374.

Levine, C. "The Loneliness of the Long-Term Caregiver." *New England Journal of Medicine* 340 (1999): 1587–1590.

Levine, I., and B. Rubiner. "Caring Across the Miles." *Better Homes and Gardens,* Apr. 2005, 194–199.

Levine, S., et al. "Home Care." *Journal of the American Medical Association* 290 (2003): 1203–1207.

Levinsky, N., et al. "Patterns of Use of Common Major Procedures in Medical Care in Older Adults." *Journal of the American Geriatrics Society* 47 (1999): 553–558.

Lewis, T. "Using the NO TEARS Tool for Medication Review." *British Medical Journal–USA* 4 (2004): 520–521.

Liao, Y., et al. "Recent Changes in the Health Status of the Older U.S. Population: Findings from the 1984 and 1994 Supplement on Aging." *Journal of the American Geriatrics Society* 49 (2001): 443–449.

Lin, O., et al. "Screening Colonoscopy in Very Elderly Patient: Prevalence of Neoplasia and Estimated Impact on Life Expectancy." *Journal of the American Medical Association* 295 (2006): 2357–2365.

Lunney, J., et al. "Patterns of Functional Decline at the End of Life." *Journal of the American Medical Association* 289 (2003): 2387–2392.

Lunney, J., et al. "Profiles of Older Medicare Decedents." *Journal of the American Geriatrics Society* 50 (2002): 1108–1112.

Lyons, W. "Delerium in Postacute and Long-Term Care." *Journal of the American Medical Directors Association* 7 (2006): 254–261.

MacLean, D. "Unhappy Families: A Closer Look and How to Help." *Caring for the Ages* 2 (2001): 6–8.

Mahady, M. "Help Wanted: Is the LTC (Long-Term Care) Nursing Shortage Improving or Getting Worse?" *Caring for the Ages* 5:1 (2004): 1.

Marziali, E., et al. "Persistent Family Concerns in Long-Term Care Settings: Meaning and Management." *Journal of the American Medical Directors Association* 7 (2006): 154–162.

Mausbach, B., et al. "Ethnicity and Time to Institutionalization of Dementia Patients: A Comparison of Latina and Caucasian Female Family Caregivers." *Journal of the American Geriatrics Society* 52 (2004): 1077–1084.

May, W. *The Physician's Covenant.* Santa Ana, CA: Westminster Press, 1983.

McCaffrey, M. "Yours, Mine, and Heirs." *New York Times,* Dec. 8, 2005.

McCormick, W., and P. Boling. "Multimorbidity and a Comprehensive Medicare Care-Coordination Benefit." *Journal of the American Geriatrics Society* 53 (2005): 2227–2228.

McNicoll, L., et al. "One-Year Outcomes Following Delirium in Older ICU Patients." *American Geriatrics Society Annual Meeting 2004 Paper Abstracts,* S2.

Miller, J. *The Caregiver's Book: Caring for Another; Caring for Yourself.* Minneapolis, MN: Augsberg, 1993.

Miller, K., et al. "The Geriatric Patient: A Systematic Approach to Maintaining Health." *American Family Physician* 61 (2000): 1089–1104.

Min, L., et al. "Predictors of Overall Quality of Care Provided to Vulnerable Older People." *Journal of the American Geriatrics Society* 53 (2005): 1705–1711.

Mitchell, S. "Financial Incentives for Placing Feeding Tubes in Nursing Home Residents with Advanced Dementia." *Journal of the American Geriatrics Society* 51 (2003): 129–131.

Mitchell, S., et al. "Clinical and Organizational Factors Associated with Feeding Tube Use Among Nursing Home Residents with Advanced Cognitive Impairment." *Journal of the American Medical Association* 290 (2003): 73–80.

Murray, S., et al. "Illness Trajectories and Palliative Care." *British Medical Journal–USA* 5 (2005): 287–292.

Narayanan, S., et al. "Change in Disease Prevalence Documented in Minimum Data Set (MDS): Four-Year Trends in Nursing Home Admissions." *Gerontological Society of America Annual Meeting 2005 Paper Abstracts,* 657.

National Alliance for Caregiving and AARP. *Caregiving in the U.S.* Washington, DC, 2004.

O'Connor, P. "Adding Value to Evidence-Based Clinical Guidelines." *Journal of the American Medical Association* 294 (2005): 741–743.

Oliver, D., et al. "End-of-Life Care in U.S. Nursing Homes: Review of the Evidence." *Journal of the American Medical Directors Association* 6 (2005): S21–S30.

Parrish, J. "An Unquiet Death." *Journal of the American Medical Association* 296 (2006): 2531–2532.

Penrod, J., and J. Hupcey. "Family Caregiving at the End-of-Life." *Gerontological Society of American Annual Meeting 2004 Paper Abstracts,* 302.

Pettey, S. "Report Recommends Standards for Assisted Living." *Caring for the Ages* 4:6 (2003).

Post, S., et al. "The Real-World Ethics of Dementia." Special issue, *Annals of Long-Term Care* 7 (1999): 7–11.

Pronovost, P., et al. "Medication Reconciliation: A Practical Tool to Reduce the Risk of Medication Errors." *Journal of Critical Care* 18 (2003): 201–205.

Pynoos, J. "The Future of Housing and Residential Care for Older Persons." *Annals of Long-Term Care* 7 (1999): 144–148.

Rabow, M., et al. "Supporting Family Caregivers at the End of Life: 'They Don't Know What They Don't Know.' " *Journal of the American Medical Association* 291 (2004): 483–491.

Rastas, S., et al. "Association Between Blood Pressure and Survival over 9 Years in a General Population Aged 85 and Older." *Journal of the American Geriatrics Society* 54 (2006): 912–918.

Rector, T., et al. "Pneumonia in Nursing Home Residents: Factors Associated with In-Home Care of EverCare Enrollees." *Journal of the American Geriatrics Society* 53 (2005): 472–477.

Ricauda, N., et al. "Home Hospitalization Service for Acute Uncomplicated First Ischemic Stroke in Elderly Patients: A Randomized Trial." *Journal of the American Geriatrics Society* 52 (2004): 278–283.

Rice, B. "Should You See Nursing Home Patients?" *Medical Economics,* May 6, 2005.

Roger, V., et al. "Trends in Heart Failure Incidence and Survival in a Community-Based Population." *Journal of the American Medical Association* 292 (2004): 344–350.

Rosen, S., and N. Weintraub. "The Efficacy of Performing Screening Mammograms in the Frail Elderly Population." *Journal of the American Medical Directors Association* 7 (2006): 230–233.

Sassoon, S. "When I'm Alone." In *The Heart's Journey,* London: Heinemann, 1928.

Satish, S., et al. "The Relationship Between Blood Pressure and Mortality in the Oldest Old." *Journal of the American Geriatrics Society* 49 (2001): 367–374.

Schols, J., and A. de Veer. "Information Exchange Between General Practitioner and Nursing Home Physician in the Netherlands." *Journal of the American Medical Directors Association* 6 (2005): 219–225.

Schumacher, J. "Examining the Physician's Role with Assisted Living Residents." *Journal of the American Medical Directors Association* 6 (2006): 377–382.

Schumacher, J., et al. "Physician Care in Assisted Living: A Qualitative Study." *Journal of the American Medical Directors Association* 6 (2005): 34–41.

Shakespeare, W. *As You Like It.* Pelican edition. Ed. Frances E. Dolan. New York: Penguin, 2000.

Shield, R., et al. "Physicians Missing in Action: Family Perspectives on Physician and Staffing Problems in End-of-Life Care in the Nursing Home." *Journal of the American Geriatrics Society* 53 (2005): 1651–1657.

Somogyi-Zalud, E., et al. "The Use of Life-Sustaining Treatments in Hospitalized Persons Aged 80 and Older." *Journal of the American Geriatrics Society* 50 (2002): 930–934.

Steel, K., and T. F. Williams. "It's Time to March." *Journal of the American Geriatrics Society* 54 (2006): 1142–1143.

Stone, D. *Reframing Home Health Care Policy.* Cambridge, MA: Radcliffe Public Policy Center, 2000.

———. "Physician Involvement in Long-Term Care: Bridging the Medical and Social Models." *Journal of the American Medical Directors Association* 7 (2006): 460–466.

———. *Long-Term Care for the Elderly with Disabilities: Current Policy, Emerging Trends, and Implications for the Twenty-First Century.* New York: Milbank Memorial Fund, 2000.

Stone, R. *In the Next Galaxy.* Port Townsend, WA: Copper Canyon Press, 2002.

Supiano, K., et al. "Mobilizing Frail Nursing Facility Residents, Families, and Resources to Facilitate Return to Community Living." *Gerontological Society of America Annual Meeting 2005 Paper Abstracts,* 101.

Tanaka, K., T. Takahashi, Y. Mochizuki, D. Ichikawa, and K. Ogasawara. *The Ballad of Narayama.* VHS. Directed by Keisuke Kinoshita. New York: Kino Video, 2000.

Tagore, R. *The Gardener.* New York: Macmillan: 1913.

———. *The Gardener.* Whitefish, MT: Kessinger Publishing Company, 2004.

Teri, L. "Improving Care for Older Adults with Depression and Cognitive Impairment: Advance in Nonpharmacological Treatments." Presentation, Forum on Aging, University of Vermont, Burlington, VT, May 26, 2005.

Thomas, E., and T. Brennan. "Incidence and Type of Preventable Adverse Events in Elderly Patients: Population-Based Review of Medical Records." *British Medical Journal* 320 (2000): 741–744.

Thomas, L. "Effective Dyspnea Management Strategies Identified by Elders with End-Stage COPD (Chronic Obstructive Pulmonary Disease)." *Gerontological Society of America Annual Meeting 2005 Paper Abstracts,* 123.

Tilden, V., et al. "Out-of-Hospital Death: Advance Care Planning, Decedent Symptoms, and Caregiver Burden." *Journal of the American Geriatrics Society* 52 (2004): 532–539.

Tulsky, J. "Beyond Advance Directives: Importance of Communication Skills at the End of Life." *Journal of the American Medical Association* 294 (2005): 359–365.

Twersky, J., and H. Hoenig. "Rehabilitation." *Clinical Geriatrics* 9 (2001): 20–33.

U.S. Dept. of Health and Human Services. Agency for Healthcare Research and Quality and the Centers for Disease Control. "Physical Activity and Older Americans: Benefits and Strategies." 2002. http://www.ahrq.gov/ppip/activity.htm.

U.S. Dept. of Health and Human Services. National Institute on Aging. *So Far Away: Twenty Questions for Long-Distance Caregivers.* Bethesda, MD: U.S. Government Printing Office, 2006.

———. *Talking with Your Doctor: A Guide for Older People.* NIH Publication No. 05-3452. Bethesda, MD: U.S. Government Printing Office, 2005.

U.S. Dept. of Health and Human Services. National Vital Statistics System. *United States Life Tables, 2002.* National Vital Statistics Reports 53:6. Hyattsville, MD: National Center for Health Statistics, 2004.

Walston, J., et al. "Research Agenda for Frailty in Older Adults: Towards a Better Understanding of Physiology and Etiology: Summary from the American Geriatrics Society/National Institute on Aging Research Conference on Frailty in Older Adults." *Journal of the American Geriatrics Society* 54 (2006): 991–1001.

Wasserman, J. *Shaping the Future of Long-Term Care and Independent Living—2005–2015.* Waterbury: Vermont Dept. of Aging and Independent Living, 2006.

Weisbart, E. "Safer Prescribing for Older Adults: Clinical and Business Imperatives Aligned." *Clinical Geriatrics* 14 (2006): 18–24.

Welch, H., et al. "What's Making Us Sick Is an Epidemic of Diagnoses." *New York Times,* Jan. 2, 2007.

Whalen, J. "Britain Stirs Outcry by Weighing Benefits of Drugs Versus Price." *Wall Street Journal,* Nov. 22, 2005.

White, V. "Old Age Is a Disease of Inactivity: A Statistical Interpretation of the Senior Olympics." *Geezerjock,* Aug.–Sept. 2006.

Williams, M., et al. "The Short-Term Effect of Interdisciplinary Medication Review on Function and Cost in Ambulatory Elderly People." *Journal of the American Geriatrics Society* 52 (2004): 93–98.

Winakur, J. "What Are We Going to Do with Dad?" *Health Affairs* 24 (2005): 1064–1072.

Winn, P., and A. Dentino. "Quality Palliative Care in Long-Term Care Settings." *Journal of the American Medical Directors Association* 5 (2004): 197–206.

Winzelberg, G., et al. "Beyond Autonomy: Diversifying End-of-Life Decision-Making Approaches to Serve Patients and Families." *Journal of the American Geriatrics Society* 53 (2005): 1046–1050.

Woolf, S. "Pseudodisease." *British Medical Journal–USA* 3 (2003): 178.

Zarowitz, B., et al. "The Application of Evidence-Based Principles of Care in Older Persons (Issue 3): Management of Diabetes Mellitus." *Journal of the American Medical Directors Association* 7 (2006): 234–240.

Acknowledgments

A core group of family and friends have helped me to transform "talk" into the written word. First was my dear friend Deming Holleran, who teased some of these ideas out of me years ago for an educational project. In the time since, her commitment to helping me bring my ideas and experience to the public never flagged. Our daughter Kate, the Great Communicator, offered regular moral support by telephone and e-mail and threw herself into her grandmother's care when crisis arose. Close friend and novelist Barbara Dimmick, was a steady supporter and guide, encouraging me to discover myself through the written word. My medical colleagues, Dr. Dale Gephart and Joanne Sandberg-Cook, Geriatric Nurse Practitioner, understand the world of elder care as well as anyone I know. Conversations with them gave me the confidence to tell this story of the late-life journey. A friend through decades of sharing, Nancy Perkins, recognized the value of an early manuscript and had the golden touch to bring it to the attention of the larger publishing world. My agents, Richard Pine and Carrie Cook of Inkwell Management and Nestegg Productions, helped me recognize my audience and refocus the writing. Finally, Gail Winston, my editor, with her fine intuitive connection with the subject, drew out of me greater depth of human content and understanding and edited and re-edited the text so carefully and thoughtfully. Her able assistant Sarah Whitman-Salkin responded to my regular queries and concerns instantly and thoughtfully.

Through the many years of writing, my mother, Bertha, opened up her own personal story as she never had before and always asked "how the book was coming along," even when delirium was robbing her of her orientation. Throughout my life she has been my most steadfast supporter—"both on the court and off," my friends would add. Over the last decade, my sister Maureen joined hands with me in a wonderfully faithful and coordinated effort of caring.

The list of those who contributed to my mother's well-being is village-length. The senior living community of Arbor Green supported Bertha for nearly twenty years, never once suggesting she was too frail to stay. Drs. Dewald, Imm, and Shebuski kept their covenant with her. Friends Fran Harmala and Hazel Tepsa stepped in for nearly two years to prop her up with daily visitations and care. Portage View Hospital, Stillwaters Assisted Living Center, the Visiting Nurse Association of Vermont and New Hampshire, the Keweenaw Home Nursing and Hospice, the Houghton County Medical Care Facility, and the Omega House residential hospice were formal helpers during her journey, their staffs comforting both her and our family. Pastors Jimalee Jones and Susan Odegard and the congregation of Gloria Dei Lutheran Church were committed supporters of our family to the end.

In many ways while writing this book, I feel I have simply been the mouthpiece for the many patients and families I have had the privilege to care for over many decades. As do many doctors, I learned so much from their shared lives as well as their shared problems. Here I would include those I worked with in the many small communities of the Upper Valley region of Vermont and New Hampshire. The people of the small impoverished island of Carriacou, Grenada, West Indies taught me more about the inherent resiliency of human beings than a lifetime of practice in the United States could have. The residents and staff at Kendal-at-Hanover, where I served as medical director, gave me the opportunity to create a medical service based on my belief in human resilience and the wisdom of aging and try to incorporate both into good health care and caring. Several colleagues and friends from Kendal deserve special mention for their help and inspiration—medical partners Drs. Walter Frey and Julie Fago, who helped me "in the trenches," and Joanne Sandberg-Cook, whose clinical acumen and emphasis on establishing mutual trust with patients and families was foundational to our shared enterprise. Kendal residents Dr. Tom Almy, Jim and Carol Armstrong, Professor Fred Berthold, Walter Frank, Edie Gieg, Dr. Barbara Gilbert, Connie and Fred Landmann, and Jack Moorhead, were friends and wise counsel over many years.

When I felt daunted, a group of writer-friends encouraged me and taught me about "the writing life"—Fred Dillon, Brian Fitzpatrick, Sonja Hakala, Henry Homeyer, Cynthia Huntington, Gary Lenhart, Cleopatra Mathis, Robert Nichols, Grace Paley, Bill Phillips, Clyde Watson, Carol Westberg, and Barbara Yoder. A number of other people read parts or all of various drafts of this work and offered useful feedback: Nancy Baker, Dr. Steve Bartels, Dr. Ira Byock, Dr. Edward Campion, Rev. Katie Crane, Dr. Linda Emanuel, Dr. Daniel Federman, Patrick Flood, Professor Ray Hall, Dr. Brian Hennen, Rev. Doug Moore, Daniel Perry, Peter and Keenie Richardson, Bob Riessen, Lisa Taylor, Dr. Dan Tobin, Dr. Maurice Woods, and Doris Yates.

The Department of Community and Family Medicine at Dartmouth Medical School supported me and this project throughout: my friend and department chairman, Michael Zubkoff, and colleagues Laurie Harding, Mimi Simpson and Drs. Chris Allen, Nan Cochran, Elliott Fisher, Don Kollisch, Tom Parrot, Jim Strickler, and Phillip Wade, and staff members Sandi Cragin and Darlene Howe. Additionally, the Community Geriatric Group—a diverse group of faculty physicians, nurses, nurse practitioners, and administrators—deserve thanks for their participation in many hours of early morning discussions of geriatric care which lent stories and substance to this book. The statistical expertise of Chuck Townsend and Craig Westling of the Dartmouth-Hitchcock Medical Center helped me to understand how health systems performed for elders. Special thanks also to Dr. Patricia Blanchette and her staff for supporting my brief visit and work on this project in the Geriatrics Department at the University of Hawaii. And thanks to the Windsor County Medicaid Waiver Team for including me in their team meetings.

Sections of this book were written at peaceful locations which allowed some insulation from daily chores and for this I thank Dinny Adams, David Binger, Romer Holleran, Jim and Ann Moore, Bob Moran, Lisa Taylor, and Ethel Woolverton.

Financial support for the work and time to write came partially from a most generous grant from the Dosoris Fund of the Upper Valley Community Foundation, a regional division of the New Hampshire Charitable Foundation and the Vermont Community Foundation. Special thanks to Lisa Cashdan and Kevin Peterson for their personal interest in my work.

Early in my project, I received much encouragement from many people in regaining my own health. For this I thank especially Bill Ciofreddi, my physical therapist, and Leonardo, my personal trainer in Playa del Carmen, Gordon Bower, and my many Playa friends.

Not because they supported less, but because they fit no special category are many other friends who contributed anecdotes and stories, not all of which could be included in the book, but which enhanced my understanding of families. Although I will undoubtedly fail to mention someone, let me here thank Joan Angelis, John Arata, John and Jamie Bemis, Jan Binger, Dr. Bruce Bocking, Sally Bower, Darby and Liisa Bradley, Ames Byrd, Linda Genovese, Louise Hamlin, Sandy Harris, Larry and Rainie Kelly, Tom and Paula Keltner, Beth Krusi, Norman Levy, Judy Music, Rosemary Orgren, Dr. Worth Parker, Francie Prosser, Nancy Tehan, and John Vogel.

Past mentors of enormous importance to my development as a physician are Dr. Herman Lisco, my late friend and former dean at Harvard Medical School, Dr. Hugh Bower, my original practice partner, and family physician educators Drs. John Frey, Joe Morrissy, Dick Walton, and Ian MacWhinney.

Finally, this book could not have been written without the loving support of my wife and writing partner, Pamela Harrison, who started by encouraging me to write in order to heal and who continued to help me to find my voice by often knowing it better than I did myself. Many of the stylistic elements in the book are attributable to her poetic sensibility, which took my ideas and experience and transformed them into much more readable narrative. All who know both of us will recognize her beautiful touch.

Index